UNLEASHING KETAMINE

THE PIONEERING PSYCHEDELIC THERAPY RESHAPING MODERN MEDICINE

FRANK M LIGONS

Foreword by
JOHN NEWMARK

Frank M. Ligons, MS
Foreword by John Newmark, MS, LPC

The information in this book is based on the author's research and personal and professional experiences. It is not intended as a substitute for consulting with your physician or other healthcare provider. Any attempt to diagnose and treat an illness should only be made under the direction of a healthcare professional.

The publisher and author do not advocate using any particular healthcare protocol but believe the information in this book should be available to the public. They are not responsible for any adverse effects or consequences resulting from using the ideas or procedures discussed in this book. Should the reader have any questions, they must consult a professional healthcare advisor.

ISBN: 978-1-7368925-6-5 (paperback)

978-1-7368925-5-8 (ebook)

978-1-7368925-7-2 (downloadable audio file)

978-1-7368925-8-9 (hardcover)

Unleashing Ketamine: The Pioneering Psychedelic Therapy Transforming Modern Medicine

Next Gen Medical, LLC

139 East Main Street

#735

Carnegie, PA 15106

info@FindKetamine.com

Editor: Jim Davis

Proofreading: Shelly Davis

BONUS MATERIALS

IMPORTANT NEWS: Why did I switch to At-Home Ketamine therapy after five years of IV treatments?

I explain everything in this video: FindKetamine.com/AtHome.

Are you a candidate for at-home ketamine treatments?

Have you heard about "bad trips" on ketamine? Otherwise known as "k-holes," these experiences can be intense and unsettling. Not everyone experiences k holes. But they can make for a wild ride. But don't worry. You'll make it through!

Please enjoy your bonuses by visiting FindKetamine.com/BookVideos.

Don't miss this shocking video!

DEDICATION

To my sister, Marcie, who plays all of her roles (mother, wife, daughter, aunt, niece, cousin, and colleague) so well. You're an inspiration.

UPDATES

Information updates are available at *FindKetamine.com*.

Hi, this is Frank Ligons here. Thanks very much for reading. I present both live and virtually to audiences in need of hope and facts about this life-changing, breakthrough treatment. Please tell me how I can help you and your organization by scheduling a call at *FindKetamine.com/bookfrank*.

Thank you!

FOREWORD

John Newmark is a Licensed Professional Counselor (LPC) with a Master of Science (MS) degree. For over twenty years, his counseling has improved his clients' ability to function and thrive.

Using a cognitive-oriented approach, he helps liberate sufferers of mental health disorders related to anxiety, depression, trauma, and relationship dynamics. He also teaches others about these conditions and the techniques he finds successful in treating them.

Mr. Newmark currently serves the areas surrounding Washington, D. C., through his private practice in Alexandria, VA. He provides ketamine-assisted therapy through this location.

October 2023

Ketamine opens up a whole new way of seeing the world. Its dissociative effects help patients recognize the difference between their distressing thoughts and reality. When this happens, they experience freedom from taking their mental world too seriously. Consequently, their mood is frequently lifted, and even lifelong anxiety disorders can become much more manageable.

I have patients who have been on antidepressants and benzodiazepines for years. Some go on to discover much deeper relief through ketamine treatment. Ketamine shows them how everything is connected. That realization can impart a profound sense of safety that anxiety sufferers rarely experience.

For those in treatment for depression or anxiety who are still unable to feel joy, consider ketamine therapy. Its efficacy rate is higher than virtually every other approach. Plus, the side effects are usually minimal.

Ketamine research efforts are expanding, and study data continues to improve. While treatment is currently expensive, that will soon change.

Working together with ketamine's astonishing ability to facilitate breakthroughs is very gratifying and gives me great hope for the future treatment of mental health conditions.

John Newmark, MS, LPC

JohnNewmark.com

INTRODUCTION

Dear Reader,

If you feel desperate, helpless, and hopeless, I get it. Those words describe my battle with depression over the past twenty-five-plus years.

Can you guess when those feelings ended? After my first ketamine treatment.

Don't get me wrong. I still grapple with bipolar disorder and obsessive-compulsive disorder. But since I found ketamine therapy, I haven't lived with the crushing despair that consumed half of my life. With a bit of that weight lifted, I can envision the possibility of a brighter future.

My hope is that this book will set you on a similar path of success.

Most sincerely,

Frank M. Ligons

1

DANGER AHEAD!

When I finished my undergraduate studies, I entered the job hunt believing wholeheartedly that money solved everything. When it came time to apply for a position, whichever route offered the most money and elite credentials was the way for me. If you've lived chasing fame and fortune, you know that can fuel depression.

In my case, I chose a career in management consulting for a "Big 5" firm. Large paychecks began arriving every two weeks. And I welcomed them! Exorbitant Lexus lease payments didn't keep from splurging on my dream car. My designer wardrobe had me feeling suave and sophisticated. Top-shelf liquors were now in reach.

Believe me, I'm not bragging. Those were all things I enjoyed, for sure. But my mental health challenges were making a huge dent in whatever happiness I expected. Like many before me, I discovered how reaching fantastic financial milestones became hollow destinations. I'm a member of that club.

Medications were prescribed. They made me tired—sufficiently so that I'd show up for work two hours late every day. Do you know how you feel when you show up two hours late? Nervous. Nervous about being yelled at and potentially losing your job.

Within a couple of years, I found myself calling in sick frequently. Eventually, I hit the wall and contacted Human Resources, explaining that I required medical leave. That's an embarrassing phone call to make when you're twenty-three years old. Plus, I was fearful of the angry calls I expected to flood in from my superiors.

Medical leave carried me until it was clear I would not be coming back, ever.

I'm not sure what we would label what happened to me today; terms are constantly changing. But I'd call it a nervous break-down. I couldn't function. I was mired in a constant stew of sadness and fear. This lapse into disability would happen several more times. The medications were poor at quelling my symptoms, but they excelled at inducing weight gain and extreme fatigue.

An entire year passed as I was locked in my house alone–too terrified to leave. More doctors. More meds.

I tried the "Attacking Anxiety" course by Lucinda Basset I had seen advertised on TV every 15 minutes. The course was a massive box of audiotapes. I began listening to them and practicing the exercises.

Over time I worked up to venturing outside for thirty-minute walks each day. The tapes taught me that I wasn't a "freak." Men and women of every age suffer from severe anxiety and depression. That comforted me. Plus, I learned relaxation routines. Ultimately, I started to internalize these protocols to help me face panic attacks. About a year after having to leave work, the tapes' lessons prepared me to stand up and work toward restoring my life. Thanks, Lucinda!

Salvaging the wreckage of my prior life wasn't easy. Before leaving my consulting job at twenty-three, I had begun investing in real estate–purchasing and renovating. Unfortunately, I lost those gains during my prolonged medical leave and plunged into bankruptcy by twenty-four.

People talk down to people who've declared bankruptcy. The truth is that most declarations in the U.S. are due to ruinous medical situations. Regardless, it was embarrassing.

My mother and I visited an attorney. I clearly recall fearing that he wouldn't believe me. By that, I mean my disabling condition wasn't visible. I wasn't disfigured, limping, or wrapped in bandages; I looked "normal." My anxious mind imagined this lawyer thinking: Why is this "normal-looking" young guy filing for bankruptcy? The last thing I wanted was to feel judged for my fall from working life. Looking back, I was already doing an excellent job of judging myself. If you've ever been sidelined by a medical issue, you know how much self-blame can come with that. It's easy to beat up on yourself for taking "too long" to recover and needing to "try harder".

Little did I know then that this boom and bust pattern driven by health challenges would continue throughout my life.

At some point, I developed suicidal thoughts. And, while life delivered its ups and downs, these dark thoughts remained steady.

And so it went, on and on, year after year. Boom and bust, chased by menacing clouds of terror and overwhelm.

In 2010, I was on the rebound from a period of disability and looking for a new way to be productive. At that time, the field of biomedical informatics was really hitting its stride. The University of Pittsburgh's medical school had a department specializing in this field, and Drs. Wendy Chapman and Rebecca Jacobson gave me a doctoral fellowship to fund my education. I prayed for a healthy run.

Biomedical informatics, as its name suggests, isn't the easiest program. You must pass numerous classes in challenging topics such as machine learning, Bayesian statistics, advanced calculus, and scientific programming in Python. And this doesn't include the specific medical knowledge required to apply these classes to real-world problems in medicine.

I'm sure many people in the University of Pittsburgh Medical School's Department of Biomedical Informatics were more intelligent than I. Most of my classmates already had graduate-level degrees– Master's, PhDs, and MDs. Some had several. Maybe they didn't find our courses hard. But I did. Especially statistics. Ugh. Statistics. Great professors. Torturous material.

The strain of taking classes and publishing in academic journals cranked up my stress levels. With that came more intense depression and anxiety. Those, in turn, began driving me into isolation. Isolation brought sadness.

Meanwhile, my OCD engine was running 1,000 miles per hour. The thought of getting less than an "A" in any of my classes frightened me. Even when my advisors repeatedly reminded me that the program's purpose was much less about these classes *per se*, and much more about collaborating, publishing, and presenting novel research, my obsessive mind wouldn't let go. Sure, I got my "A's," but I felt like I took ten years off of my life doing it. Still, I was making some progress.

While riding this boom of opportunity and productivity, I should've known that a big bust was coming. Four years into my Ph.D., I came down with a puzzling set of symptoms. First, there was memory loss. Not like an "Oh, I can't remember the name of my first-grade teacher," memory loss. But an "I can't remember what I said only 30 seconds ago" memory loss. Sounds funny in retrospect. However, there was one group that did not find it humorous: my academic advisory committee.

I don't blame them. I was in graduate school and not functioning. That wasn't acceptable. Plus, at the time, no one understood the reason for my forgetful, slipshod behavior. From their perspective, I just wasn't bringing my A-game.

People think being a professor is a dream job. It might be for some. But it's unspeakably challenging. Talk about putting in the hours: conducting research, publishing papers, requesting grant money, teaching classes, and mentoring students is ceaselessly demanding. Understanding their workload explains why during our weekly meetings, my absurd lack of progress rubbed them the wrong way.

These busy PhDs and MDs were setting aside time to usher me into my own graduate degree. Repaying them by ignoring their suggestions and showing up dull-witted must have been infuriating. They likely thought I was suffering from a lousy attitude rather than a severe illness. While the origin of my cognitive deficits remained unknown, appearing at these meetings and observing my committee's irritation fed my anxiety and exacerbated my condition.

It wasn't until later that the real cause of my slippage emerged as a rare, potentially lethal, neurodegenerative disease.

Before the mystery unravelled things got worse. Much worse. By the time I "woke up," I was three months into a stay in a psychiatric hospital—psychotic, erratic, and devolving from unknown causes.

2

MY DRINKING BUDDY BARACK

FAST FOOD CONTAINS A LOT OF PRESERVATIVES. BUT NOT ENOUGH TO remain consumable after two weeks in the back seat of my car in the hot summer sun. Apparently, I spent some time prior to my hospitalization picking up food from McDonald's, Wendy's, and Panera, tossing it in my back seat, and driving around until I was hungry.

Kanye West and I have never collaborated on an album. Yet, for a few months, I was positive that we had. Yep, I'd call him up from the mental hospital and discuss the details of our soon-to-be-released project.

President Barack Obama and I never hashed out the topography of the geopolitical landscape over beers. But for a few months, I swore he was my world-wise drinking buddy.

Bathrooms are for relieving oneself. But for a few months, I peed in the trash can in the room of a fellow patient. If you're wondering, she was actually rather gracious about it.

I had been through emotional collapses before. But this time, falling into disability included forgetting how to eat, toilet, shower, and communicate. My mental health complaints flipped from feeling too stuck in my mind to completely losing hold of it. My downward trajectory was sharp and swift.

Unfortunately, it took a long time for my physicians to puzzle out my diagnosis. By the time I "awoke" from psychosis, a season had passed. It was a warm summer when my symptoms began, but I emerged from months of amnesia into a chilly fall. A glance out of my reinforced plexiglass hospital window clued me in.

Time was running out when we discovered that my affliction was Hashimoto's encephalitis, a rare autoimmune disorder that attacks the brain. My cluster of devastating symptoms included profound, instantaneous memory loss, difficulty with speech, and inability to perform daily tasks such as feeding myself, dressing correctly, and carrying out routine functions like placing a phone call or taking a shower.

Amid all this, I began keeping a journal describing the hair-raising, unforeseeable twists and turns I encountered. If you are interested in reading this page-turner, subscribe to my newsletter and I'll keep you posted: *FindKetamine.com/updateme*.

To make a VERY long story short, it took two years to recover from that mind-boggling ordeal. Given my brain damage, I could not finish my Ph.D. Thankfully, I did graduate with my Master of Science.

On top of the OCD and depression that began in my teens, suicidal thoughts were wearing me down. All of this started before the encephalitis and continued after, leaving me in no condition to work.

For one thing, I required traumatic brain injury therapy to relearn how to count. Then, there was stumbling through writing and sending emails. These were on top of the dozens of physicians I met with over those years treating everything from blood clots to peeing the bed.

My bipolar disorder and OCD anchored me to a shifty pier in a foggy port. So, while rebuilding my brain and body, I kept my eyes peeled for treatments to help my longstanding mental health conditions.

Four years later, I caught a break. My sister told me about a novel treatment option for depression called ketamine therapy.

Like most people, I didn't know ketamine was the world's most common anesthetic. I only heard it was a "club drug" and an animal tranquilizer. Upon further research, I discovered that this safe and affordable medication, when administered in small doses, could relieve treatment-resistant depression and perhaps help with bipolar and OCD.

As a detail-minded person with a medical background, I was cautiously excited. A whole year of research elapsed between the time my sister told me about it and my decision to have my first ketamine therapy session. That journey of learning about ketamine, deciding to try it, and my initial experiences are covered in my previous book: *IV Ketamine Infusions for Depression: Why I Tried It, What It's Like, and If It Worked.*

This astonishing procedure stopped my twenty-five years of suicidal thoughts in their tracks! That was over three years ago, and while I receive monthly boosters, those dark thoughts rarely return.

That's why I wrote my first book: to spread the good news to people who need hope and help. It is available as an eBook, paperback, and audiobook at Amazon and all major retailers. Thank you to everyone who supported that project, which debuted as a #1 Amazon New Seller, topping the Amazon charts in several categories, and earning Honorable Mentions from The *Bookfest Book Awards* and The *Firebird Book Awards*.

The book is simple, easy to read, and step-by-step. It's a must-have for sufferers of treatment-resistant depression and essential reading if you are considering Ketamine for you or a loved one. You can purchase signed copies and bulk orders at *FindKetamine.com*.

Ketamine flipped the switch for me–from someone plagued by thoughts of death to showing others a way out. I'm only one of many with this life-saving testimonial. Many people, through ketamine and other new therapies, find themselves leading fulfilling lives on the other side of epic life struggles.

3

WHY YOU SHOULDN'T GIVE UP

No one has ever contacted me with a complaint about ketamine or questioned my successful journey with it. If people are arguing against ketamine's potential, they aren't sending me that feedback. This doesn't mean that ketamine is a cure-all. What it does mean is that at least some previously desperate patients are now benefitting from this therapy.

Everything I've heard in the past few years has further fueled my optimism about this treatment. Ketamine continues to alleviate hard-to-treat mental health conditions, severe pain, and substance abuse. The scope of clinical research into ketamine is blossoming. Long gone are the days of a "handful of studies." Now, it's difficult to keep up with all of them.

Conversations about ketamine are now everywhere. I hope to answer your questions and spark new ones. I don't know it all, but I'll get you started down the road of knowledge and encourage you to learn more about this breakthrough treatment. You can continue your education at *FindKetamine.com*.

4

BACK TO BASICS

KETAMINE IS A SEDATIVE-HYPNOTIC WITH PAIN-RELIEVING EFFECTS. IT is commonly used as an anesthetic. When used for surgery, it keeps the patient asleep, paralyzes the muscles, mitigates the pain response, and "disconnects" the mind from the body. Ketamine is also technically a psychedelic, though not a typical one like LSD, psilocybin, and ayahuasca.

Before ketamine came into use in the 1960s, phencyclidine—better known as PCP or angel dust—was used to sedate patients for surgery. But emergence from that sleep was not always prompt and safe. Some patients suffered psychotic spells and depression that could take days or weeks to resolve. Ketamine grew out of the need for an agent similar in function but with a faster, more predictable, and safer "emergence."

Phencyclidine testing on animals revealed the desirable anesthetic markers of psychological detachment, muscle relaxation, and temporary paralysis. Despite this, misgivings remained concerning its application to humans because of its propensity to induce erratic delirium. Dramatic descriptions of this side effect often appeared on the news, with PCP users exhibiting "super-human strength" while impervious to pain. They were described as psychotic, delusional, paranoid, and predisposed to violence. Reports of "deranged" suspects undaunted by law enforcement became mainstays of sensational nightly news footage.

Because phencyclidine could produce such behavioral extremes, ketamine's ability to provide similar anesthetic benefits, albeit with fewer and less concerning adverse effects, was met with enthusiasm.

Ketamine's use dates back to the 1960s as a battlefield medicine, used to rescue injured soldiers from shock, trauma, and cardiovascular collapse from blood loss.

In a variety of wartime scenarios, ketamine:

1. keeps the body immobile and stable during operations.

2. relieves pain from injuries and the surgery required to repair them.

3. sustains patients in mortal danger from blood loss. One side effect is acute hypertension. Elevations in pressure and pulse may be significant. However, when a patient is losing blood, these hemodynamic side effects become benefits, maintaining pressure despite losses in volume.

4. imparts amnesia around traumatic events, be it surgery or other painful experiences.

5. is short-acting, with the patient returning to consciousness quickly.

6. is less likely to produce "emergence syndrome" than its predecessor, phencyclidine.

7. does not require temperature-controlled storage.

Ketamine's uses addressed in this book are mostly low-dose intravenous infusions administered in outpatient clinics that range from small, with a handful of employees, to large, with multiple locations, treatment rooms, and staff.

Emergency departments use ketamine for intense pain relief, sedation, psychiatric stabilization, and preservation of cardiovascular integrity during blood loss.

Ketamine is also used in low-resource settings worldwide, where access to safe, effective, and inexpensive anesthetics are absolutely essential.

5

MORE THAN AN ANESTHETIC

KETAMINE HAS BEEN AN INVALUABLE ANESTHETIC WITH FDA approval since 1970.

Most of its other uses are not explicitly FDA-approved. Still, all medical professionals with a license to write prescriptions are legally permitted to prescribe ketamine "off-label" for a medical need outside of its officially-approved purpose.

Ketamine is frequently prescribed off-label because its many uses fall outside that of an anesthetic. The permission to utilize pharmaceutical benefits without the constraint of the initial drug-approval process equips clinicians with more treatment options. This practice is legal and common. As many as one in five prescriptions are for off-label purposes.

Alongside its expanding medical use, ketamine also became known as the party drug "Special K." It gained notoriety for attracting recreational users drawn by its euphoric dissociative effects, particularly in dance clubs.

In 2019, ketamine's "mirror" molecule, esketamine, was approved by the FDA for treatment-resistant depression.

The brand name of esketamine is Spravato; it's a nasal spray, not an infusion.

There are some differences between esketamine and ketamine. While ketamine infusions are legal when prescribed by licensed physicians, the FDA has not explicitly approved them to treat depression and other conditions. On the other hand, where first-line treatments have failed, esketamine is approved for use when combined with an antidepressant in patients with treatment-resistant depression and suicidal thoughts.

Many medical professionals agree that ketamine has potential beyond its historical uses. Because of its long track record, ketamine's safety parameters are well-understood. However, those applications (anesthesia, pain relief, and shock from injury) are usually limited to one session, unlike ketamine treatments for depression, and other mental health conditions, that require repeated treatments over the long term. Less is known about ketamine's safety in these scenarios. The long-term effects of periodic treatments in these contexts need time to manifest.

6

FINDING TREATMENT

CHOOSING MEDICAL CARE IS ONE OF LIFE'S MOST IMPORTANT decisions. Therefore, determining which ketamine clinic is best for you is worth careful consideration.

The number of clinics continues to expand across the U.S. and is spreading into Europe and other continents. With its consistent success record, access is becoming more readily available. That's why the *FindKetamine.com Clinic Directory* enables you to search for ketamine clinics worldwide.

Ketamine treatment usually requires some form of consultation. Its goal is to determine if you are a good candidate, formulate a treatment plan, and answer any questions so you can make an informed decision before moving forward. Even though ketamine is generally safe, a review of your medical and psychiatric history is necessary.

7

WHAT EXPERTS AND PATIENTS SAY

In the four years that I've been a ketamine patient, I'm continually awed by how many people report improvement. For some people, that's a break from emotional anguish. For others, it's a respite from unrelenting pain. Some substance abuse sufferers are finally escaping relapse and making substantial progress toward remaining drug-free.

Various types of clinicians are on the front lines overseeing the thousands of breakthroughs fueling the ketamine therapy movement. I sent questions to several prominent practitioners. Here are their written replies:

Dr. Glen Z. Brooks — Founder of New York Ketamine. Pioneer who established one of the first clinics offering low-dose ketamine infusions for mental health conditions. Has administered thousands of such treatments.

Q: What types of patients are most likely to experience relief from ketamine therapy?

A: There are two "best predictors" of which patients are most likely to respond to ketamine.

The first is the story, i.e., the patient had a difficult childhood, maybe, but not necessarily, physical or sexual abuse. Other problems often heard are growing up with parental fighting or divorce leading to insecurities and fears of abandonment. Additional examples are cases of parental substance abuse, domestic violence, hypercritical and controlling parents, or narcissistic parents displaying no emotional positivity or nurturing. For other patients, it might be problems at school, such as bullying, isolation, low self-esteem, struggles with gender identity, body dysmorphia, racial discrimination, or religious bigotry. These can all lead to childhood stress or trauma.

The second is age. Ketamine facilitates synaptogenic-neuroplastic repair. Younger brains are more neuroplastic, with success rates approaching 75 percent. The benefits of this neuroplasticity drop off quickly, with patients older than seventy seeing success rates no higher than 50 percent.

Q: What do you find most encouraging about the advances in ketamine therapy?

A: What is most encouraging is the fact that our patients are considered otherwise treatment-resistant, meaning that they have not responded to traditional psychiatric meds, psychotherapy, or in some cases, hospitalization and electroconvulsive therapy. A large percentage have suicidal ideations. Even with this degree of impairment, the success rates with ketamine infusion therapy are encouraging and impressive.

Q: Is this revolutionary therapy becoming more available to those who need it?

A: When I started our center in Manhattan in 2012, there were only eight infusion centers nationwide. Now, there are more than four hundred. So, geographically, ketamine is widely available. There are issues with the cost of treatment since insurance plans rarely cover ketamine therapy.

Many centers offer reduced fees for financial hardship, veterans, and first responders.

Dr. Henry Macler - Founder of Pittsburgh Ketamine. Highest honors in medical school and psychiatric rotations. Former chief resident in anesthesia at Harvard. Has administered thousands of ketamine treatments.

Q: Having treated more than 600 patients with over 4,000 treatment sessions, what stands out about your clinical experiences?

A: The therapeutic experience involves the patient's level of consciousness approaching and including disassociation. There is often a pleasurable sense of great comfort to the patient during the treatment.

It seems essential to help the patient feel as safe and relaxed as possible BEFORE the treatment begins. Having the close presence of a trusted mate or friend at the bedside, or a hug and hand-holding, can assist.

Particularly in the case of a patient's first treatment, there is a natural anxiety about the unknown. With the help of their companion, the patient can verbalize these concerns and enjoy the reassurance through something even as simple as a gentle squeeze of the hand. Some patients engage in soothing conversation with their companions.

Q: How would you describe the thoughts and feelings of patients during the treatment?

A: Some patients perceive themselves as floating on a rapidly moving stream. Others "hear" a steady, monotone sound. Regardless of the manifestation, having someone nearby can be calming.

Q: Do the effects of treatments accumulate?

A: An enormous sense of safety and joy tends to accumulate with successive treatments. Wholesome emotions like these are significant because many patients have not had these feelings in everyday life, in a long time, or ever.

During the treatment, changes in the patient occur at a cellular level. We hope the impact of these changes over successive treatments will persist for significant periods. (As a patient, these changes have positively affected my personality over the long-term.)

Q: How does ketamine adjust one's emotional sensitivity?

A: Ketamine patients may feel an increased perceptivity to the feelings of others and how others feel toward them. This effect can be immensely positive in establishing and preserving a sense of well-being for the patient.

Q: You have prior experience with applying electro-convulsive therapy to patients with depression. What is your current thinking on comparing electro-convulsive therapy to ketamine as an intervention for depression?

A: I would undoubtedly recommend ketamine for depression rather than electro-convulsive therapy. There is no loss of memory and very minimal cardiovascular risk.

Q: How would you advise a potential ketamine patient to proceed?

A: There is no substitute for an informed patient and a well-practiced clinician.

I also contacted ketamine patients to share their experiences. Here are their replies through our correspondence:

Terah Kuykendall - Female, 40s, Texas.

Q: How did you come to use ketamine therapy?

A: Migraine disease reared its ugly head when I was fifteen. In the beginning, the migraine attacks were few and far between. They slowly progressed in frequency until 2006, when I "earned" the diagnosis of chronic DAILY migraines. My disease continued to get uglier, necessitating my leaving a much-loved career at Coca-Cola and going on disability in 2011.

Q: Had you tried many things before ketamine?

A: For twenty-plus years, I went through over forty medications and a dozen neurologists in several cities. In late 2012, I FINALLY received a referral to a neurologist and headache specialist who had been local all along. (Yes, surprisingly, a neurologist and a headache specialist are two separate things. Less than five hundred neurologists in the U.S. are certified headache specialists!)

My new doctor was excellent about "believing me" regarding all of the meds and procedures I'd previously tried. (Sadly, in the migraine community, most doctors will start you all over again, almost as though those meds will suddenly work now that you're under THEIR care.)

Q: How did you first learn about ketamine?

A: My new doctor spent about a year ensuring I had all of my I's dotted and T's crossed. Then, one day in late 2013, she asked if I wanted to try ketamine.

Q: What was your initial impression?

A: "The horse tranquilizer?" I've learned that's pretty much everyone's standard reply!

Q: What were your concerns?

A: Honestly, I went into it with my only concern being that ketamine would be just one more thing that didn't work. I was in such constant and agonizing pain place that I was willing to do everything my new doctor suggested.

Q: How did you find the information that convinced you to try it?

A: I didn't. It was 2013, and there was literally nothing available to research. Even worse, merely mentioning "ketamine," even today, elicits negative, judgmental reactions from most people.

I used Facebook to create the public page "Ketamine for Chronic Migraine" and the private group, "Medical Ketamine for the Treatment of Chronic Migraine." Both have over one thousand followers. The private group tightly controls anonymity. This privacy allows chronic migraineurs to communicate, ask questions, and draw support from fellow sufferers without "family drama" and social criticism.

Q: Did you have difficulty getting the treatment?

A: Initially? No. My neuro had to prove I would still fail with an intravenous treatment called DHE (typically one of the final treatment options) to "prove" that it (still) did not help me. I was admitted to the hospital overnight for that but then hooked up to ketamine the next day. I'm not sure why, but the hospitals here will only provide ketamine in their intensive care units, even for low doses.

Once we determined what schedule and dosing worked best for me, I would go into the hospital for three days of IV ketamine.

Q: Why did you preface that answer with "initially?" What stood in your way?

A: Insurance got in the way, and, as we all know, that's their standard operating procedure. Insurance would no longer cover inpatient ketamine infusions. Infusions changed into outpatient procedures. Finding any kind of ketamine provider is difficult enough. This alteration added to the list of impediments to receiving treatment.

Q: What form did you use (intravenous, intramuscular, sublingual)? How did you choose it?

A: I have always received ketamine intravenously. How did I choose that? Well, as I mentioned earlier, there was simply no information out there at all. I didn't know there were different forms of the drug. Therefore, I went along with what the doctor prescribed. What's the frustrating saying, "I didn't know what I didn't know"?

Q: Did the treatment experience differ from your expectations?

A: I knew the first ketamine infusion dosing would start small and increase over several days in the hospital. So, I took a cross-stitch project, some books, snacks, and drinks in a little cooler—my "creature comforts."

Let me just say that while being infused with ketamine, you cannot see straight. You can't focus. There are at least three of everything. That blew all of my time-fillers straight out of the window. So, for what turned out to be a ten-day stay in the hospital, I did nothing but keep my eyes closed and listen to TV reruns of NCIS Los Angeles!

Interestingly, sound during an infusion remains easily understood. For me, it becomes more focused and very intense. Many infusion patients I know will listen to music or YouTube videos. Maybe because I'm a musician, I find any music with a steady rhythm too intense. Instead, I listen to Native American flute albums.

The one thing I despise in an infusion setting is hearing a song I know. I get overwhelmingly "stuck" in it. The best thing for me has been a free app called MyNoise. It has all of the typical ambient and relaxing sound options. I use the white noise setting. It's especially awesome because the white noise is completely customizable. For example, if my head is in a horrible pain place, I can turn up the lower frequencies and decrease the highs. Plus, it helps block out the constant infernal beeping of all the monitors and machines!

I want to clarify that my ten-day stay in the hospital for a ketamine infusion is not at all typical, I promise! The Jefferson Headache Clinic (I believe it's in Philadelphia) has a five-day inpatient protocol. Still, after that initial stay, I would remain an inpatient for three days. An admission for a multiple-day visit is usually only implemented for very high-dose (cumulative) ketamine sessions.

Q: What was your treatment plan? Frequent intervals and then less frequent?

A: My initial most effective inpatient treatment plan was "Let's see how you do!" I would start feeling worse between the eight-to-ten-week mark, so I'd schedule to go back in.

With outpatient infusions, insurance has now mandated four consecutive days per month. These are at a significantly higher dosing rate per hour but across only a few hours. This change makes the ketamine experience considerably different from the slow-drip variety.

However, my cumulative dose is less than half of what I would receive as an inpatient. This reduced dose has cut my period of relief in half. Plus, getting transportation when you are only allowed to be picked up by close friends or family is exceedingly challenging to arrange. It's gone from dropping me off at the hospital on Monday morning and picking me up Wednesday night to back and forth across town for drop off and then again for pickup across each of four days.

Scheduling rides is now one of my worst sources of constant stress. I must be cognizant to avoid bringing that tension into my infusion. I agree with my fellow patients that it is crucial to enter the ketamine infusion peacefully, with a sense of calm and as much serenity as you can muster.

Q: How long before you noticed an improvement?

A: I had a terrible hangover the first week after my initial infusion and was so discouraged that another last-ditch treatment had failed again. But I noticed a difference at the start of the second week. A very impressive difference!

My average daily pain levels decreased. The frequency of the more severe migraine attacks and their duration both decreased. Ketamine's ability to increase the efficacy of my migraine abortive rescue medications is still an astounding concept for me. Of course, I welcome it with open arms.

Q: Have the improvements increased, stayed the same, or decreased over time?

A: The improvements I had in the beginning have decreased over time. But this is not due to the efficacy of ketamine. It's due to reducing the dosage strength.

The transition from inpatient to outpatient has made a huge difference, but in the wrong ways. The cumulative dose of a four-day outpatient infusion was half that of a three-day inpatient infusion. The sessions also shifted from being inpatient under the purview of my neurologist to outpatient infusions with a pain-management specialist.

There was another decrease when I transferred care to a different doctor. Then, yet another significant reduction in dosing came when clinical ketamine guidelines (for treating pain, NOT MENTAL HEALTH) were published by the American Society of Regional Anesthesia and Pain Medicine in 2018.

Ketamine has already proven itself to me. I hate knowing that a proven-to-work treatment exists but is no longer available. It is absolutely incomprehensible to me how a physician could settle for my lost quality of life. Alas, here and now, I simply cannot access ketamine at an adequate dosage level anymore. I'm sure you can tell this is more than just one of my "soapboxes." My entire life has been negatively affected by the diminished treatment.

Q: What's your long-term treatment plan?

A: Honestly? I have no clue. And I have to admit, I don't have a positive outlook on it.

Q: Have you been recommending ketamine since your treatment began?

A: Back on a happier subject? Yes, I constantly recommend ketamine for treating chronic migraine disease, especially when it's a struggle to make it through to the end of every day. Sometimes, I'll bring it up to another chronic pain patient looking for treatment options. However, any expertise I might have is limited to migraine disease.

Q: What would you say to someone considering ketamine?

A: Please, please, please look into just the possibility of adding ketamine to the tools you have in your shed for fighting your disease. However, I personally choose to mention two huge caveats:

First, while more and more information is becoming available online for your ketamine research, it can be extremely difficult to identify what is legitimate research versus a sales pitch by a ketamine provider. I do not trust any information about ketamine posted online by practices looking to attract more patients. This is a good reason not to trust what you read!

They will tout their "proprietary ketamine treatment" as the absolute best available ketamine treatment option. Then, you read further and see that their accompanying treatment medications (for anxiety or nausea) are identical to everywhere else.

Second, when researching ketamine and discussing it with others, remember that no one person is "right." (And isn't that just a terrible way to approach a potential new treatment option?) Every patient and physician is different.

This means that every individual's treatment protocol may vary. One of the rules in my Facebook group is that people must use auxiliary verb terminology, such as "should," "could," and "might," etc., in their posts/comments. When someone says that another person's doctor/protocol is wrong, many freak out, and it can be challenging to unruffle everyone's feathers.

Q: Are there any tips for patients seeking to get the most from their therapy?

A: By the time you are researching ketamine, you are, unfortunately, part of a select group of patients who have been very sick for a very long time. That's why I say:

Be open to trying anything and everything.

Be open to trying ketamine more than once. Give the medication a proper chance before determining (with your doctor) that it doesn't work for you or that any side effects outweigh the benefits.

Ketamine is only one tool. You have a lot of other implements in your tool shed that you must not just put by the wayside–other medications, nutrition, depression meds, or therapy. You cannot go into ketamine treatment thinking it will be your treatment to end all treatments. It's not. So, in your desperate desire to improve things, try not to make things worse!

Q: What is your approach or insight into payment or insurance?

A: Your doctor is responsible for proving you've been down a long road of failing treatment. So, you must have a transparent relationship with them and the ability to discuss exactly what their paperwork says. There is a high probability that the paperwork your provider submitted to your insurance doesn't convey the urgency with which you present and discuss in your appointments. I have had too many neurologists complete paperwork talking in generalities about my headaches when I have a legitimate and specific diagnosis of chronic migraine disease.

Appeal, appeal, appeal. Don't settle for one and done. Your insurance provider has multiple levels of appeal escalation available. Plus, you can also appeal to your state's insurance division. My neurologist initially suggested doing that because it seems to light a fire under the insurance company for coverage approval. I once had my insurance suddenly disapprove of a rescue medication I had been taking successfully for many years. When I got to the point where I appealed to the Texas State Division of Insurance, that medication was approved in three days.

Consider keeping detailed lists and logs that support your claim. Do you keep a pain journal? What about which medications you take and the pertinent dates of each? (Yes, your doctor should include failed meds in their initial request for coverage authorization, but you would be surprised how often that doesn't happen. Either you or your doctor must document failed treatments. Sadly, it might have to be you.)

Do you keep records of non-medication treatments like massage or physical therapy? A mental health provider may be willing to write a statement on your behalf.

Include copies of any relevant published papers or studies that support your position.

All of the above also rings true when applying for and appealing denials of Social Security Disability Income. Qualifying for this assistance program requires that you demonstrate mental difficulties along with your physical disabilities. I guarantee the side effects of most of your medications include confusion, inability to focus, etc.

Take advantage of your insurance's out-of-network coverage. If you can get an itemized bill from your provider and submit it along with your insurance company's out-of-network claim form, you might be reimbursed for a percentage of that claim. This may exceed 50 percent, depending on your particular insurance.

An additional approach to paying for medical treatment is to take advantage of any employer-sponsored health savings account available to you or your spouse. These accounts serve two critical roles. First, the money placed on that card is income that cannot be taxed, freeing up those monies for additional medical expenditures. Second, the account is fully funded for the entire year at the beginning of that year. Yes, you will have the applicable payroll deductions throughout the whole year. But this might be the only thing that can get you through that horrible period of reset annual deductibles.

Q: What do you expect will be the future of ketamine treatment?

A: It's a mixed bag...

PROS:

Studies are only now beginning to bear out the successful application of ketamine treatment.

Ketamine is becoming more widely known and accepted by physicians as a treatment for acute and chronic pain and mental health.

CONS:

In just the past few years, there has been a sudden influx of ketamine "pop-up" clinics. These are typically the providers who are advertising their sales pitch as fact. It is absolutely 100 percent necessary that the doctor you choose to administer your ketamine treatment has actually been trained in how to administer ketamine. According to the American Society of Regional Anesthesia and Pain Medicine guidelines, these are "anesthesiologists, critical-care-trained physicians, and pain physicians." A potential ketamine patient simply must do their due diligence.

I worry that inadequately trained providers will make mistakes. Not only will these be detrimental (even potentially deadly) to the patient, but they will quickly negate any positive trajectory ketamine has gained as a treatment for chronic pain.

The instant stigma of ketamine as a "horse tranquilizer" and recreational drug is foremost in people's minds when the "k word" is mentioned.

Unfortunately, you (the patient) must educate yourself to combat the cynicism of "horrified" friends and family. Is ketamine used in veterinary practice? Sure. But it's been FDA-approved FOR HUMANS as an anesthetic since the 1960s. And, while it is a controlled substance, it is NOT a narcotic. Keep in mind it is the most widely used anesthetic on the planet.

Q: What do you find most reassuring about your ketamine journey?

A: It exists. It works. Given a high enough dose, it will work for me again. Now if I could just get back there.

Sherry Jo Matt - Female, 50s, Pennsylvania. Founder of the Stop the Judgment Project

Q: Is ketamine safe?

A: Yes! Absolutely! I would encourage anyone who is considering ketamine treatment to do it! If you are thinking about it for yourself or your loved one, there is a reason for your interest, and I believe it will help! I wish I had done it years ago for myself and my daughter's addiction/substance use disorder.

Q: How did it work for you?

A: I'll be as blunt and as honest as I can. Ketamine SAVED MY LIFE! I was in a very dark place after my daughter died from a fentanyl drug overdose at twenty-one years old. I didn't know how dark my mindset was until I got help. I didn't have a suicide plan; I just did not want to be here. I didn't think I was contributing to anyone or anything. I was circling the drain.

After my treatments, I am now seeing the light again. I am now feeling a reason to get up. I am currently looking forward to my life with my husband and son. I can't bring my daughter back! However, I can let my son have a mother who is present. A mother who is alert and living! A positive mother. A mother who cares.

Q: What is the ketamine treatment like?

A: Well, for my center in Florida, it was an IV drip. It was fifty minutes. It was administered by a professionally trained staff of nurses and with a doctor present. It was much like a doctor's office. It was a controlled setting. I felt VERY SAFE!! Never once did I feel uncomfortable. I met with a professionally accredited counselor many times during my three-week visit. I am still in contact with the clinic.

Q: What did you try before ketamine?

A: Everything!!! That is a long list. For example: therapy, yoga, wine, antidepressants, and Reiki (a Japanese form of energy healing). Looking back, I was depressed for several years leading up to my daughter's death. When dealing with an addicted loved one, it is very difficult to get them help. You watch them suffer. You see the magnitude of pain they are in. It hurts so much. It is very hard to separate your love, logic, and concern while competing with their love of drugs and the hold those drugs have on them.

Q: How would you advise someone requiring similar help?

A: So, let's be honest and forthright about this. I was in a lot of pain watching drugs kill my daughter. We both circled the drain—me slowly dying while watching her slip away. I watched Siena dying from street drugs that changed and shifted her in ways no parent wants to see. Those drugs led to her death.

When she died of an overdose, I wanted NOTHING to do with drugs. When ketamine was first suggested to me for therapy, it was an adamant "NO WAY!!!! Drugs killed my daughter." I wanted NOTHING to do with more drugs. I was not having anything to do with "getting high" and "going on a trip." My mindset was, "I am a fifty-eight-year-old suburban mom living in an affluent area. I don't do drugs! I did not do them through high school or college. Why would I start now, especially after 'drugs' killed my daughter?"

After many conversations with the clinic, they told me this treatment was different. This was a controlled environment. This was medically prescribed. This is proven to help others. Very carefully administered. A physician friend reassured me of its safety–such a low "micro" dose.

I was also told that I wouldn't forget my daughter through the process. However, I would be "disassociating from the pain."

When I reflect on it now, Siena did die of substance abuse disorder. However, her mental health struggles with bipolar and borderline personality disorder drove her drug problem. I firmly believe that ketamine can help with substance abuse and various mental health conditions, including those my daughter confronted.

My conviction to bring awareness to the possibilities of ketamine therapy as applied to substance use disorder and mental health challenges culminated in the foundation of the Stop the Judgment Project: *StopTheJudgement.org*.

Ellen D'argenzio — Female, 30s, Maryland.

Q: Is ketamine safe?

A: I believe this will have to be established by each individual's doctor. During my treatments, I was monitored by a nurse, a doctor, and a blood pressure cuff. So, yes, I felt very safe and comfortable. I was also honest about my anxiety, about anything that might make me hallucinate. So, they started me off slowly.

Q: How did ketamine therapy help you?

A: It worked miracles for me. It's really hard to explain. Anything I had repressed for months, and even years, and felt guilty about came out during my treatments. For instance, we had to make a really hard decision to put my cat to sleep. She was a rescue cat shuffled from home to home before she came to live with us for six happy years.

However, the vets couldn't figure out what was wrong with her toward the end. Thousands of dollars later and a cat with blood in her urine, we decided to put her to sleep. I felt really guilty about this because we didn't have definitive answers. During my third ketamine infusion, I saw my Ellie (kitty) with her sister Annie (golden retriever), who passed away from cancer two years earlier. They were playing together in heaven. I cried during my infusion, but I needed to see them move on. My mind and body must have known this.

I hope that explained a little about what it was like. The physical aspect of the feeling of ketamine is feeling "a little out of it." Once finished, I felt extremely clear and sharp with tons of energy.

Q: What did you try before ketamine?

A: Before I tried ketamine, I had tried pretty much every common antidepressant. I am still on a low dose of Cymbalta to keep the depression at bay because the ketamine infusions were expensive.

Q: What would you recommend to someone looking for help?

A: If someone struggles to function normally in everyday life like I was, I recommend calling the insurance company and working with their psychiatrist if nothing else has worked for them. I am a huge advocate for this treatment, and it's a shame that such an inexpensive drug costs $450 an infusion. I also think insurance should cover it without you having to jump through so many hoops. I was one of the fortunate ones who was able to afford it.

Anonymous — Male, 30s.

Q: Is ketamine safe?

A: From my research and personal experience, ketamine is an incredibly safe drug that is frequently used and well-understood.

Q: How did it work for you?

A: Ketamine allowed me to disconnect from my emotions entirely–to focus on real issues, real acceptance, and a real understanding of life beyond my current circumstances.

Q: What is the ketamine treatment like?

A: It is an intravenous treatment, so you are hooked up to an IV. That mechanism administers the drug. They may add Zofran to prevent nausea.

The ketamine dose is calibrated depending on your weight and previous drug use experience. It is then dispensed evenly over forty minutes. Once the drug affects your system, you will feel a sense of calm, floating, and comfort that increases over the treatment's duration. If you want to amplify those feelings, you can close your eyes. Keeping your eyes open or listening to podcasts or music will ground you and lessen the dissociation.

Q: What did you try before you found ketamine?

A: Multiple antidepressants, benzodiazepines, psilocybin, alcohol, histamine blockers, beta-blockers, and marijuana.

Q: How would you advise someone with a similar situation?

A: This safe treatment will allow you to experience a breakthrough of profound peace and understanding. It may help you to perceive things differently going forward, which is critical in managing or resolving mental health issues such as depression.

Anonymous — Male, 20s.

Q: As someone who has used ketamine recreationally, what would you like people to know about your experiences?

A: I've only had a handful of experiences as I have a hard time finding ketamine (without a prescription). However, I had profound experiences with the substance, and I'd be very happy to share my experiences with you.

People have it all wrong about drugs being inherently bad. They're just physiological/psychological tools, if you ask me.

Q: I'm eager to hear more of your thoughts. Readers might appreciate ideas and experiences about ketamine they don't usually hear about. They only hear from doctors and official sources. Yet, many people are interested in what someone outside the medical industry reports. Do you have any notes from ketamine trips to give us insight into your experiences?

A: Yes, I have messages and notes about things I wrote and conversations I had. These may help you understand my perspective while on the drug.

Transcript of a conversation between Anonymous and one of their friends follows:

Bro, I'm not pressuring you. I just want to explain what it's like. It is very different from psychedelics. It's a dissociative class drug, and it is extremely difficult to have a bad experience because your ego has almost no effect on the experience. It's not an intense, introspective roller coaster of whirlwind emotions and insanity like LSD or psilocybin. It's very strange but peaceful. You take on the mood of your environment.

It feels very good to the body, like you're so utterly relaxed and experiencing this liquid feeling. You just move so easily (low dose, mind you. Heavy dose, you just lie there with your eyes closed and can barely move), and I find it awesome. It's like the pleasurable aspects of a psychedelic without the intensity or emotional properties.

I'm in a state of pure understanding and connectivity to everything right now. And I just wanted to say that you two are my best friends in the world, and I love you guys so much. I want to say an infinite number of things to you guys about how much your friendship means to me and how great I think you are. But, man, you guys just rule. I often wonder what you guys think of me, but I know it is with love, so it doesn't bother me. Love you guys.

I had 1.4 grams that night and did it incrementally in 50, 100, and 200 mg doses, for reference.

Q: It sounds like "K" helps you be more expressive of your feelings. Does it always affect you like that? Or do you sometimes feel negative emotions?

A: K most certainly helps me be more expressive. In all the times I've done it, it's always been very similar. I've never for even a millisecond felt a tinge of negative emotion while high on it, either. But I have heard some stories of people freaking out.

Q: It sounds like you've been able to keep the dose low enough to prevent the "k-hole."

A: I chose to because, as we've talked about, I research any substance I will consume beforehand. I memorized what the typical dosages are and their effects. I was very curious about the different levels of the experience. I started low, doing 70-80 mg. bumps one night. Then, I waited a week for my tolerance to reset. Finally, I went for the white whale and sniffed 500 mg., and went into a deep oceanic hole. I can't remember anything from that session except the physical sensation, which felt like I was in water, made of slime, and tossed to and fro.

I didn't black out during it, but I just can't remember much of anything. With smaller dosages, I remember basically the whole thing.

From what I've read, anything inhaled over 100 mg. has the potential to k-hole somebody.

Q: What dose have you settled on? It's one thing to get 100 mg. dripped over a forty-minute session. Taking a "bump" is totally different.

A: What do you mean by "settled on?" As in my preferred? 70 mg.-90 mg. is my sweet spot. That's where I get all that boosted awareness, empathy, and a sense of more accurately using my language to express my thoughts.

I've always been wary of injecting drugs because I've seen the worst. But ketamine is one I'd consider trying because of its low addictive potential. And I could imagine how much better it must be with such a notable difference in bioavailability.

I'm not as familiar with the descriptions of the different levels of ketamine dosages as I am with the classic psychedelics. I hear "anesthetized," and I assume "catatonic," like just immobile. But if returning from the "trip" without memory of the experience signals anesthetization, then definitely. That 500 mg. dose I did is very scrambled in my memory, and I only vaguely recall a few details.

8

'WHY ARE YOU TRYING THIS STUFF?'

BECAUSE PSYCHEDELIC THERAPY CARRIES AN UNJUSTIFIED STIGMA, you may feel uncomfortable explaining this treatment choice to loved ones and physicians. People look down on it even though they rarely know much about the topic.

Below are some tips for answering questions that establish clear and productive lines of communication:

Q. What is ketamine therapy?

A. It's complex and cannot be summed up in a few sentences. Your family may need to do a bit of reading (or listening) to understand the basics. Consider giving them a copy of *IV Ketamine Infusions for Depression: Why I Tried It, What It's Like, and If It Worked*. It will provide quick, easy-to-understand answers to most questions.

Q. Why do you seek ketamine therapy?

A. Close family and friends probably know about your diagnosis and how it impacts your life. They have seen you suffer, cry, hide, and go to doctor after doctor. Hopefully, they'll understand that if infusions of ketamine may help you, you are willing to investigate. There is no harm in figuring out your options with licensed medical personnel guiding you. In general, proactive patients get better outcomes.

Many patients come to ketamine when they have run out of options. They have bounced around the medical system without results–trying various medications and undergoing multiple therapies. Even patients who feel better are often concerned about the side effects of their treatments and continue seeking better options.

It's no surprise when someone suffering from a problematic condition confers with their doctor about ketamine therapy. If your physician determines that ketamine is safe and potentially helpful for you, it may be worth considering.

Q. Why ketamine for mental health particularly?

A. Most people have heard of common psychiatric drugs like antidepressants. Drugs such as Prozac, Paxil, and Lexapro are well-known because of advertising and widespread use. Of course, there are many lesser-known drug classes. There are also such non-pharmacological treatments as electroconvulsive therapy, hypnotherapy, biofeedback, and meditation.

People in your life may ask, "With all of this 'normal' stuff available, why are you trying this weird ketamine option?"

The answer is that ketamine sessions may help where these other approaches have not. This therapy may not be well-known, but it certainly has a positive reputation among the thousands of people benefitting from its use.

Q. How do I help my family understand?

A. It can be hard to explain your condition. Some, such as migraines, Chron's disease, or cancer, may be more comprehendible. But many health difficulties involving emotional and physical pain that create functional limitations are rarely experienced by the general public.

When the rigors of your illness are impossible to communicate, your desperation to find relief may be also. How often has someone told you to "take a pill" or "get over it"? If only it were that easy.

A medical affliction can leave you literally screaming for a cure. If and when people around you understand that, they will realize your need to try anything your doctor deems worthy of consideration. If that choice is difficult to understand, seems drastic, or ill-advised, you can ask your doctor to explain the situation by taking your family/friend/advocate with you on your office visit.

Q. What if my family pushes back?

A. Ultimately, the answer to that question comes down to you. If you are a minor or unable to pay for treatment, your options for overcoming these roadblocks may be limited. But never give up. Talk to your doctors or other loved ones, friends, and sources of support. Find safe people: school counselors, support groups, or church members.

Most importantly, stay safe. Tell people if you are thinking of hurting yourself or others. Keep the suicide hotline on you, just in case. You also have 911 at your disposal.

If, as an adult, you can coordinate treatment with your provider and possess the financial wherewithal, you may have to make an uncomfortable decision, on your own. Remember, you're the one with the disease. And, unless your decision-making is impaired, you and your medical team need to do what is best for you.

Q. What if my doctor is not supportive?

A. Finding out if ketamine may be a good treatment option for you must be determined through discussions with physicians. You can start with your own and consult others as necessary. Considering all of your treatment options is essential. In these modern times, various approaches to dealing with illnesses exist. Ketamine is just one possibility—and a legitimate one.

One unique aspect of the ketamine approach is that many physicians do not consider it risky for most patients. Its long history demonstrates an impressive record of safety.

What happens if your doctor—someone you've been seeing for years—is not familiar with ketamine treatment? Or worse, what if they are skeptical or even against it?

Remember that no one doctor knows everything. Just think of the nearly unlimited spectrum of interventions: medications, surgery, nutrition, traditional Chinese medicine, Ayurveda, cold therapy, hot therapy, and so many more. How can one person stay abreast of absolutely everything in their field?

Yes, doctors must complete a certain amount of ongoing education. And, yes, most are eager to find safer and more effective treatments for their patients.

Still, everyone has limits on their time and attention.

So, inquiring as to your physician's familiarity with ketamine treatments is not personal nor unprofessional. When you think about it, it's very unlikely that anyone would know much about this. Awareness of ketamine is growing in the medical and public spheres. But it's far from universal.

Q. How do I proceed?

A. You could follow these steps:

1. Get your ketamine education. That could be at *Findketamine.com*, along with specialists in your illness and ketamine practitioners. Being well-informed puts you on the path to wise medical decisions.

2. Bring up ketamine with your doctor. Tell them you are wondering whether it may help your condition. Offer to direct them to the source of your information. Your physician may appreciate it.

3. Prepare for possible reactions, which may include a) they've heard of it, b) know of its success, c) are unfamiliar with it, or d) are against it.

4. Avoid arguing with your doctor. There is no need to convince them either way. As with any medical consultation, you can always seek additional opinions. Meeting with an experienced ketamine practitioner, or a specialist in your condition, are both sensible options.

5. Keep in mind that physicians who offer ketamine treatments can legally prescribe them. However, they may suggest, or even require, that you coordinate care with the approval of the rest of your medical team.

9

WHAT TO EXPECT

A KETAMINE INFUSION INVOLVES INJECTING LIQUID KETAMINE INTO the bloodstream via an intravenous needle. Nasal spray applications involve sniffing the medication through an applicator.

Preparing for an intravenous infusion of ketamine is simple. After you've found a satisfactory clinic, there are just a few things to address:

1. Get a good night's sleep. You may fall asleep during your treatment, but it's good to go into the experience rested and calm.

2. Try to avoid drama, stressful situations, and confrontations.

3. Follow the clinic's instructions governing your consumption of medications, food, and drink. They may tell you to alter your medication schedule or refrain from food and drink. It's essential to adhere to their instructions.

4. When planning your clinic visit, make sure to include time for the intake and exit procedures. Those break down into roughly

twenty minutes for intake (unless it is your first treatment, which may be considerably longer), vitals, and IV insertion, forty minutes for the infusion, and thirty minutes for reawakening.

Ketamine dosages consider several factors. At least initially, the dominant variable is the patient's weight. Most people begin at a standard weight-calibrated dose that may increase over successive sessions.

Depending on the condition being treated, the dose, and other factors, the duration of the actual infusion may vary. However, most treatments last approximately forty minutes. Treatments for pain may take much longer, up to several hours or even days.

Patients may receive Zofran and other medication to minimize dizziness or nausea.

You will sit in the treatment room, usually a quiet place with a comfortable chair and soft lighting. The staff takes your vital signs and connects the monitoring equipment–a blood pressure cuff and a pulse/oxygen clip on your finger. None of these are painful.

Ketamine comes in several forms. However, most practitioners prefer IV ketamine because the:

1) dosage can be precisely administered.

2) side effect profile is well-understood.

3) success rate and degree of relief exceed that of other forms.

A prospective vein is selected. Your skin is cleansed with an alcohol pad. The needle is inserted. Then, the hanging bag containing the liquid ketamine mixture slowly drips into your bloodstream.

Ketamine's onset is not a dramatic or frightening experience. Its effects come on gently as a deep sense of relaxation. Usually, this is quite pleasant. If a patient experiences physical or mental discomfort, the staff will intervene as necessary.

Most patients report a calm joy during the infusion. This relief from daily suffering can be truly unique! Your acute emotional or physical pain frequently diminishes during this period. As the initial anxiety passes and the symptoms of illness remit, a profound sense of escape may come over you. It is a wonderful time in the treatment.

Once the bag of ketamine runs out, the staff removes the IV and gives you time to rest and reestablish your footing. Remaining awake or drifting into sleep are both normal reactions. Either way, the beneficial effects are still imparted. Just be careful when you stand up and walk because you may be unsteady on your feet.

Post-treatment, you can expect to feel relaxed and disoriented. Sleepiness after the infusion is typical. After all, ketamine is an anesthetic.

Before leaving, patients' vital signs are reviewed and the staff asks about their treatment experience. Patient feedback will inform future treatments and confirm their readiness for clinic departure.

With respect to your treatment's results, no one can guarantee ketamine's effectiveness in all cases. However, for the spectrum of illnesses that are known to respond to this treatment, patients generally report noticeable benefits. For instance, considerable improvement has been noted in two-thirds of treatment-resistant depression cases. The odds of success for other conditions are under study.

Keep in mind that the timeframe for improvement may vary. Some patients feel better during their first treatment. Others require several before they notice any relief. Still, others never reach their desired results.

Ketamine is often referred to interchangeably with Esketamine/Spravato, but keep in mind the difference. Esketamine is the "mirror molecule," of ketamine, and is FDA-approved for treatment-resistant depression. Although closely related to ketamine chemically, esketamine is not an anesthetic. Esketamine is used intranasally, and the patient self-administers the drug under the direct supervision of a healthcare provider.

Like ketamine, esketamine may be prescribed and administered by all appropriately licensed medical practitioners, including doctors of medicine (MD), doctors of osteopathy (DO), and nurse practitioners (NP).

10

ADDICTION AND 'TRIPPING'

Low-dose IV ketamine infusions are now mainstream. Too many people are finding relief to keep ketamine's benefits secret.

When we take most medications, we don't usually expect they will make us "feel" drastically different or induce dramatic before, during, and after stages. Because ketamine is a dissociative drug, these infusions are outside of our everyday experiences. Naturally, we may have more questions and a bit of apprehension. One common concern is the potential for addiction.

As the opioid epidemic unfolds, we see the devastating effects of mass addiction. As a society, we have become sadly aware of how medication can cause a national disaster. It's frightening.

From discussions I've had with fellow patients, my impression is that concerns about becoming addicted to ketamine may be overblown. No evidence proves that medically prescribed and professionally administered ketamine treatments are addictive.

First, these infusions are given under prescribed, regulated, and carefully considered circumstances. Second, they are dosage-controlled and wear off within hours. Third, physicians providing this therapy must be licensed and carry liability insurance. Creating addicts endangers a doctor's privileges and can end their careers. Finally, patients with a history of substance abuse are carefully screened for candidacy.

Could someone with illegal, unsupervised access to ketamine (or any drug) develop an addiction? Sure. However, illicit ketamine is not widely available on the street. Nor is it a "mild" drug with the casual social appeal of alcohol or marijuana. The path to ketamine addiction requires repeated, unlawful purchases, frequent ingestion, high doses, and the absence of medical supervision.

Another concern I hear is whether one will "go crazy" or "lose their mind." Most people are inexperienced with the dissociative effects of agents like ketamine. Dissociative events, often called "trips," can take on a spectrum of descriptions from delightful to dreadful. But I've never heard of anyone suffering any long-term psychological damage from ketamine therapy.

On a related note, hallucinations are not part of my ketamine journeys, and no one has told me of experiencing them in their sessions. But that doesn't mean they don't happen. Especially if your definition is merely "seeing something that's not there."

In a way, I'm always seeing things that aren't there in these dark infusion rooms with my sunglasses on. But I wouldn't call them hallucinations. I see shapes, colors, patterns, and memories.

Psychosis is another buzzword that gets people concerned. Can ketamine induce a psychotic state?

I don't have a definitive answer from my reading on this topic. Patients with a history of psychosis are considered at higher risk for side effects, including worsening psychotic symptoms. This may exclude them from treatment. Whether someone would still benefit from ketamine therapy under these circumstances is a valid question.

Some patients experience a therapeutic return to past trauma. There are testimonials about patients "watching" past traumas, but from a disassociated distance. They are not necessarily reliving the pain of the events, but rather gaining a fresh, healing perspective.

Psychological therapy under these conditions may yield additional benefits, such as letting go of deeply ingrained emotions and thought patterns. I recently had the opportunity to receive integration therapy like this myself through an at-home ketamine treatment service. (*FindKetamine.com/bookvideos*)

Again, feeling unsure about what to expect during your infusion is totally natural and understandable. You probably don't have anything to compare it to. It's not like most things in life when someone can explain something to you by saying, "Hey, it's like that feeling when..." And that's okay because aspects of this treatment are certainly not analogous to everyday life. Still, it's a privilege to hitch a ride into a joyful place of restoration!

The vast majority of my treatments have boosted my mood, opened my mind, and flooded me with joy. On the other hand, I have undergone a few sessions that became terrifying disconnections from reality. These trips are unofficially termed "k-holes," ketamine holes, or simply "bad trips."

11

FACING THE DREADED 'K-HOLE'

K-HOLES ARE FREQUENTLY REFERRED TO AS INTENSELY DISTRESSING, frightening, or triggering experiences induced by ketamine. Confusingly, some people also refer to euphoric experiences as k-holes. But that is not the definition we will use here.

Over four years of ketamine treatment, I have experienced several k-holes, and they come in many forms. General themes include: dying, losing control of reality, being buried alive, trapped, and unable to move, breathe, or wake up.

Not everyone will confront k-holes. My impression is that for most people, most of the time, their ketamine trips are pleasant and relaxing. I'd speculate that you are especially unlikely to run into these early in your treatments when the dose is low. For myself, I did not encounter these until much later in my treatments at higher doses.

Depictions of psychedelic k-hole journeys can scare people off. The most important thing to remember is that while k-holes can be unsettling, they are not harmful.

In my sessions, I have never barreled down the tracks of a roller coaster toward a brick wall or fell head-first from the Empire State Building. Instead, the sensation of movements has been more subtle, like when my chair "reclines on its own." Even though I know it's not happening physically, this feeling is more convincing than you can imagine. In my early days of treatment, I had to double-check that I wasn't accidentally pressing the recline button on my chair. That's how convincing it was.

Rotating upside down is another common one for me. Have you seen astronauts hover and spin without an absolute sense of up or down? That's what I've felt–slow flips through space in my treatment chair. Nothing's moving fast. It's not alarming. My body doesn't start flailing or trying to rebalance itself. Despite how it sounds, it really isn't unpleasant at all. Just a bit weird the first few times. In case you're concerned, the anti-nausea medicine you're given effectively prevents your feeling ill. Even during this zero-gravity experience, I never feel dizzy, sick, or confused.

On the darker side, here are some excerpts from my k-hole journal:

Powerful experience. Sometimes frightening. I would describe it as a k-hole. Buried under rubble. Found myself rechecking if I was alive, breathing, and with my conscious awareness and control still intact.

Proprioceptive distortion, imagery, floating, turning. Slow spins, reclining back, and inclining forward.

Sunglasses blocked out the light. Headphones and music stifled all external noise. I listened to electronic dance music without lyrics from a Spotify playlist. This "ketamine kit" allowed me to disconnect my senses from the room.

The session contained periods of terrifying intensity.

I felt stuck in cosmic mud or rubble or glue. I questioned my ability to breathe. I had to take conscious breaths a few times and check my airway to ensure my tongue wasn't causing obstructive apnea. I took a sip of water during the session to reassure myself that I could swallow and breathe normally. All of my concerns were unfounded.

During a peak of terror, I reduced the intensity by temporarily removing my goggles and turning down the music. The more senses are attuned to the ordinary room around you, the easier it is to stay anchored in reality.

I'd also comment that dance music without lyrics may not be the best choice because it uses "trippy" electronic, synthesized sounds. This sonic landscape differs significantly from nature sounds or classical instrumental music.

Double vision prevents detailed interactions with my phone during the treatment. However, my headphones have a forward/backward switch to skip anything unpleasant. I highly recommend wireless headphones with this feature.

While enduring the scariest periods of the session, I remember thinking, "Whatever everyday problems or stresses I face upon waking will be easier than this helpless imprisonment." I kept reminding myself that I would soon return to the "land of the living" and regain my senses. In the meantime, I endured "hell," an unending, directionless flotation through infinite darkness, void of human contact.

I recall reassuring myself that I was still in control of the session and could discontinue whenever I wanted. Then, I would resolve to stay in, face the fears, and let them pass through my psyche. Ultimately, I knew there'd be no permanent damage.

I kept thinking there may be a benefit to allowing this fear to pass through me. I didn't want to resist or run from it. According to many experts, even distressing treatment sessions are still therapeutic. With this, I resolved to be courageous.

When setting the dosage, the doctor said he was comfortable being "aggressive" (raising the dose) because I was not near a dangerous level. He explained the large potential upside, the un-threatening downside, and the positive risk-to-reward ratio.

This higher dose presented a very noticeable elongation of the acute intoxication period. My prior session's intoxicating effects extended an hour or two post-treatment. This more aggressive therapy would require more than six to eight hours of at-home recovery. I departed the office with some stumbling, disorientation, and a bit of separation from grounded reality.

After sleeping for six hours, I felt fairly comfortable. Not extremely pleasant as I did after some treatments. Just "okay". Kind of a neutral type of intoxication. I was glad I could sleep it off and remain unstressed.

I will likely ask to repeat the same dose next time but may not use blackout goggles and such abstract music. I may go back to light sunglasses and opera.

Even in the late evening, depression did not return. I felt a bit overstimulated and restless from sleeping so much. But my mood remained bright. I didn't feel upset by family drama.

I'm looking forward to grabbing some fast food and satiating myself, even if it's unhealthy. Just glad to be alive and making strides toward improving my condition.

I'm proud to have handled the k-hole without panic. I could've unmasked myself. I could've called for help. Instead, I recognized the fear, reminded myself of the nature of dissociation, and acknowledged what it was in my own mind. I tried to use meditation techniques, but they were only moderately successful.

I hoped for a transition into bliss. It never happened, but there were moments of calm.

For me, I feel it's important to experiment within physiologically safe dosage parameters. How else would one know the therapeutic effects?

One thing is clear: I don't feel suicidal right now, and it's been approximately twelve hours since treatment.

My perception is that I was awake during the first half of the infusion and asleep during the second.

Remember thinking: I hope the afterlife is not like this.

Reminded myself that I'm in the midst of a dosage drop in one of the antidepressants I take. Went from 150 mg to 125 mg to 75 mg over the past few weeks. This may have aggravated today's journey.

I considered whether this was an out-of-body experience, like if I was hovering above my body or outside of its boundaries. I wasn't able to fully determine that. I definitely felt like there was a consciousness comprising "me" that existed outside of my body. If there wasn't, I would've been totally lost in the "buried, frozen ground," and unable to remind myself of the autonomy that would soon return after the drug wore off.

This level of immersion is not for the faint of heart. It would be very startling for someone without previous treatments under their belt. One might feel they were falling into a permanent pit, never to return. At least with some experience, you know you'll be back.

Panicking could lead to a freakout and a desire to forego future treatment. Patients must experience low-dose tranquility in their treatment

plan before entering k-hole territory. It would be a shame to forego keta-
mine's benefits due to a tough initial treatment.

As you read my notes, you might think, "That sounds dreadful!" Believe me, it was! Just keep three crucial facts in mind:

1. Whatever happens, you will not "lose your mind." You will return to normal quickly. Ketamine is a short-acting drug (one to three hours). Nothing you experience will be permanent.

2. Many clinicians believe that even uncomfortable sessions provide therapeutic benefits.

3. Your physician reviews your medical history to ensure safe treatment. You will discuss any concerns about medication interactions, psychosis, or mania and follow their licensed medical advice.

I would add that patients accustomed to dissociative states may find the treatment experience easier. For instance, patients who use alcohol or other intoxicants seem less likely to "freak out" on a ketamine trip. They "let go" more readily. People attempting to maintain strict control of their inner world might find the ketamine experience more jarring.

Most importantly, be brave. Ketamine can serve as a mysterious bridge to life-changing revelations and breakthroughs.

12

I SAW THE LIGHT

MAKING NOTES ON YOUR KETAMINE EXPERIENCES IS USEFUL. THERE are always nuggets of insight to be found in those trips. Writing things down immediately after a treatment can help. So can making an iPhone recording. You can even record yourself during the session. Just don't wait too long to listen to it because it is easy to forget the details. Similar to any time one is "drunk, high, or wasted" and "everything makes sense," that newfound comprehension often evaporates upon your return to sobriety.

Another thing that may help is jotting down the words and descriptions about your feelings during the trip. Ketamine therapy is not bound by literal, logical interpretations. On the contrary, your emotions are at least as important as your thoughts. Take note of both.

Everyone's trip is different, and you can have fascinating discussions with fellow patients about their experiences. People report just about everything you can imagine. Some patients spectate an earlier life event, and others' minds go blank as they succumb to a much-needed unwinding. Some are mesmerized by patterns of geometric light, and others stumble upon the origin of a long-held phobia. One of the best kinds of ketamine journeys clarifies a simple truth.

When life is bustling, I find it hard to concentrate. And, because of my diagnoses, my thoughts get jumbled, and my feelings can spill all over the place. Before I know it, I'm completely boggled about everything. Life is already complicated enough. Adding on mental health conditions makes it even tougher to sift through it all.

That is one reason why a ketamine therapy session is often so helpful. For instance, on one occasion, it dawned on me, more profoundly than ever before, that money isn't everything. We have all heard this a million times. But there's a difference between hearing, understanding, and internalizing.

It was truly amazing how all the cobwebs cleared away at that moment. As ketamine literally rejuvenated my brain, I relaxed in understanding that my success doesn't depend on burning myself out. Just consider, despite what I was told, and no matter how illogical, I had lived my life according to this faulty belief that money was the sole source of happiness. Suddenly, the error of my ways was laid bare. Now, this insight is deeply integrated into my being. These transformations that ketamine enables have the power to change your perspective in profoundly positive ways.

I'm no expert on psychedelic healing traditions worldwide. But I can see how these alternative states of mind facilitate new under-standings about yourself, life, and the world in which we live. Ketamine isn't just a biochemical therapy for your brain cells and nervous system. It's a psychological therapy (perhaps, even a meta-physical therapy), enhancing your insights and providing healing opportunities.

Let's summarize:

- Mild doses of ketamine induce detached tranquility. Higher doses may produce pronounced hypnotic and dissociative effects and joyful or frightening episodes.

- Some patients reprocess traumatic events or purposefully confront them. Some people revisit, relive, or re-witness prior traumatic life events. These memories can "come out of nowhere" or resurface during ketamine-assisted therapy. These episodes can result in therapeutic benefits, but when, why, and how that works is unclear.

- Experiences may differ due to many variables, including ketamine dosage and concurrent medications. If the dose is high enough (this varies among people), a person may enter a k-hole. K-hole experiences can be anxiety-provoking but not harmful.

- Your mental and emotional state upon entry into your infusion will impact the experience. For instance, when you begin your session calmly, well-rested, and optimistic, your initial sensations will likely mirror that. When I start in a good mental space, the treatment begins like a bird's smooth takeoff into the blue sky.

- Like alcohol and other substances we term "intoxicating," ketamine affects proprioception, your body's balance system that monitors your position in space, if you're moving, how fast, and in what direction. When a person is heavily intoxicated on alcohol, their proprioceptive sense is impaired, leaving them open to stumbling, bumping into things, misjudging distances, and becoming dizzy or nauseous from the distorted sense of motion. That's why you can't drive home from your treatment.

13

TIPS FOR TRANQUILITY

Now that you know a bit about the ketamine experience, here are some tips for cultivating a pleasant trip. Put yourself on the path to a pleasant session by paying attention to "set"—creating a positive mindset—and "setting," which involves the treatment surroundings and ambiance.

It is important to prepare a healthy mindset. Many substances, synthetic and natural, provide an intoxicating experience. Frequently, that experience amplifies one's current emotional state. When people are in a stressful environment or state of mind, mind-altering substances can elevate that discomfort. Conversely, entering alternative states of mind while relaxed can lead to delight.

By definition, you probably don't feel great if you require ketamine therapy. Going into therapy feeling your best is not realistic. However, you can set yourself up for success through the following:

1. Rest. Coming into treatment well-rested goes a long way. You'll feel more balanced and at ease when you've had the proper sleep. When you're tired, your body employs adrenaline to keep you awake. You may experience this adaptation as anxiety and tension.

2. Mental clarity. When you're ill, carrying around a heavy head and heart full of negative thoughts and feelings is natural. You can do a few things to combat this. Avoid disputes, distressing news media, or any other sources of unnecessary drama.

3. Food. Because you'll be on an anesthetic, your physician will instruct you regarding the rules for eating and drinking. You'll need to cease food and drink for some period before your treatment. Don't endanger yourself by ignoring the clinic's instructions.

4. Regularity. In the days leading up to treatment, try not to upset your digestive tract with unfamiliar foods. Digestive discomfort during your treatment may become distracting. I broke this rule once, making my session less enjoyable as my stomach churned and burned.

5. Medications and supplements. Be sure to follow your physician's instructions for managing your medication regimen. They may alter your schedule to maximize the impact and safety of your treatment.

6. Meditation. This need not follow a prescribed protocol. Clearing your mind through breathing, walking, prayer, or other approaches helps bring peace to your therapy. Try to leave life's worries behind.

These recommendations help put you in a good head space or mindset. That's your internal environment. The setting, conversely, includes everything happening outside of your mind–like the clinic's comforts and distractions.

Quality ketamine clinics pay attention to providing a suitable environment. A positive clinical culture is vital. Patients coming in with severe mental and physical illness are already under stress. They need care, kind treatment, and patience.

The surroundings should be quiet and comfortable. Suitable furniture, temperature, and refreshments should reinforce a sense of belonging and provision. Treatment staff must spend time with the patient to understand their unique case and concerns. Having a ketamine treatment comes with questions, especially in the beginning. An attentive clinician addresses everything the patient asks and provides answers and reassurance.

The quality of the staff that administers the treatment is critical. Considerations for a pain-free IV insertion, relaxed seating arrangement, and location of vital sign monitoring equipment are all essential. These staffers are the front line of the clinic: It's best when they present friendly, soothing demeanors.

During the ketamine treatment, the patient's environment needs protection from unnecessary sensory stimuli, including disturbing heat or cold, bright lights, startling noises, and unwanted company. Some patients would rather be left alone with minimal checkups by the staff.

Coming out from under the influence of ketamine should be gradual and unhurried. One will feel groggy and disoriented. This isn't necessarily an unpleasant experience. An excellent treatment session is pleasurable during and after. Personally, I feel great and in harmony with the world after most treatments.

Post-treatment time should include relaxing on comfortable furniture and returning home to a nurturing and serene environment. You will likely feel a sense of joy and freedom. Prolong it by planning your logistics ahead of time.

Ketamine treatment is often a great experience; it was difficult only when I ignored these tips.

14

HOW KETAMINE HELPS

As the breadth of ketamine's benefits emerges, there are more clinical trials investigating its application to an extraordinary range of scenarios:

1. Psychiatric conditions like depression, bipolar disorder, OCD, suicidal ideations, and PTSD.

2. Targeting pain-based illness is another area of promise. Many chronic, severe pain conditions are difficult to treat: fibromyalgia, chronic regional pain syndrome, migraines, and neuropathy. At the same time, the U.S. is undergoing a tragic opioid epidemic. Pain relievers with less tendency toward addiction are particularly desirable in today's medical climate. Ketamine has the potential to lessen our dependence on opioids while retaining the power to relieve pain. Ketamine may become a safer option in the analgesic toolbox. Ketamine clinics are beginning to offer pain-focused intravenous therapy for these conditions.

3. Addiction is a nationwide problem of immense proportions, spanning alcohol, an array of prescription drugs, and natural

agents such as marijuana, psilocybin, ayahuasca, and dimethyltryptamine. Opinions differ widely on the issues of legalization, personal choice, and therapeutic value. Ketamine may play a role in breaking substance abuse.

4. Diseases causing cognitive impairment, particularly in the form of dementia, are growing in number due to baby boomers' entry into later stages of life. Unfortunately, there have not been any standout successes in the treatment of this devastating illness. However, ketamine does revivify neuronal connections in the brain. Perhaps it will someday play a role in combatting cognitive decline.

Ketamine won't replace every medication and procedure. And it isn't the best treatment option for everyone. Insurance providers may continue to resist covering it. Some medical researchers may remain skeptical. Despite all of this, ketamine's impressive properties are helping patients find relief beyond their expectations.

In our Western medical system, the philosophy of highly specialized practice erodes our understanding of the body as an interconnected system. Today's medical education slices and dices the body's operations to the point where the idea of a single medication's use for many conditions sounds nonsensical. And yet, traditional medical systems with natural treatments revolve around holistic approaches in which substances impacting numerous physiological systems make perfect sense.

For example, we now know that green tea supports health in numerous ways: it's an anti-inflammatory, booster of cognitive health, fat-burning accelerant, and anti-cancer agent. Similarly, we realize that improper sleep patterns weaken the immune system, complicate weight management, and increase the chance of developing dementia in later life. These are just two examples where one arrow hits many targets. So it is with ketamine.

With the publication of more studies, the observations of more clinicians, and the torrent of testimonials, it is increasingly difficult to deny ketamine's possibilities.

Much of the current evidence explaining how ketamine works is related to the brain and nervous system.

Neurotransmitter imbalances

1. Monoamines. According to this theory, depleted levels of the neurotransmitters serotonin, dopamine, and norepinephrine cause or exacerbate the variety of illnesses addressed in this book. Antidepressants are used to restore and maintain the correct balance of these neurotransmitters. Ketamine may play a role in resetting these levels.

2. Glutamate is an excitatory neurotransmitter. Proper brain and nerve function requires the correct ratio of glutamate (excitatory) to gamma-aminobutyric acid (calming). Excess glutamate is toxic to brain cells, causing inflammation and breakdown of brain tissue. Ketamine is known for its ability to modulate glutamate pathways.

3. Gamma-aminobutyric acid (GABA). In addition to regulating the brain's level of excitement by counteracting glutamate's effects, the neurotransmitter GABA is best known as the "anti-anxiety chemical." Low GABA levels are seen in both anxious and depressed patients. Ketamine helps restore GABA levels.

4. Brain-derived neurotrophic factor (BDNF). This chemical grows and maintains healthy brain tissue, helps regulate neurotransmitter levels, and contributes to the neuroplastic processes (the "remodeling" of the brain). Ketamine increases BDNF levels.

5. Mammalian target of rapamycin (mTOR). This helps regulate the growth, maintenance, remodeling, and death of neurons.

Ketamine stimulates these pathways, promoting a healthy regulation of the neuronal cell life cycle.

6. Cholinergics. These medications act on the neurotransmitter acetylcholine. Depressive and manic episodes correlate with imbalances of acetylcholine levels in the brain. Ketamine may help modulate this balance.

Neuroinflammation

Like any other cells in the body, brain cells are vulnerable to inflammation. Microglia are brain cells with immune functions that support neurons. When microglia become activated, they trigger inflammation in the brain, accumulate high levels of quinolinic acid (a neurotoxin that accelerates neurodegeneration), and cause neurotransmitter imbalances. Research studies show that ketamine directly influences microglia, lowers the levels of toxic quinolinic acid, and protects against neuroinflammation.

Gut dysbiosis and altered gut microbiota

Once ignored by mainstream medicine, the role of the digestive system's gut flora/microbiome is now acknowledged to impact mental and physical health. Chronic stress, poor diet, and heavy antibiotic use disrupt this sophisticated system, which can lead to impairment of the immune system, systemic inflammation, and neurotransmitter dysregulation.

Altered gut flora affects the gut-brain axis–bidirectional communication between the brain and the gastrointestinal microbiome. It also increases gut permeability, activates systemic inflammation and immune responses, affects the release of neurotransmitters, harms the activity and function of the hypothalamic-pituitary-adrenal axis, and reduces brain-derived neurotrophic levels, eventually leading to depression.

Probiotics are well known for promoting healthy gut flora while inhibiting bad bacteria. Based on a systematic review of randomized controlled trials, probiotic supplementation is associated with a significant reduction in depression. Research indicates that ketamine may neutralize "bad" bacteria and support the "good."

Additional mechanisms

1. Opioid receptors. There are four different opioid receptors. Ketamine acts on all of them, explaining some of its ability to relieve pain and lower stress.

2. Cerebrovascular. Ketamine increases cerebral blood flow and metabolism.

3. Anti-oxidation. Ketamine reduces free radicals and acts to boost mitochondrial function, the energy factories in every cell.

15

WHERE KETAMINE IS NOT FDA-APPROVED

THIS SECTION AIMS NOT TO PRESENT A COMPREHENSIVE REVIEW OF the scientific literature but to offer an overview of ketamine's potential benefits.

With studies ongoing, many patients receive ketamine therapy for myriad problems "off-label." (The only exception to this is the nasal spray esketamine/Spravato. It is FDA-approved specifically for treatment-resistant depression and suicidal thoughts.)

The following list of conditions for which ketamine is not FDA-approved is not all-inclusive. Every day, this extraordinary therapy is applied to a growing variety of difficult-to-treat health challenges. They include:

Depression

Defined as a persistent state of sadness, grief, and low mood. Depression is the third leading cause of disability worldwide, affecting over 350 million individuals. Roughly one-third of people with depression suffer from the treatment-resistant form–unresponsive to the standard care model. More effective options are desperately needed.

Most prescribed antidepressants require eight to twelve weeks to provide relief–too long to intervene in suicidal patients. Intravenous ketamine infusions, on the other hand, offer a rapid and robust antidepressant effect. Maximum efficacy peaks approximately twenty-four hours after treatment, with antidepressant effects lasting one to two weeks post-infusion.

Electroconvulsive therapy is an FDA-approved treatment for depression and other conditions that do not respond to medications. It is known to be effective and provide relief before antidepressants kick in. However, ketamine can succeed where it fails and within a smaller window of time.

Suicidal thoughts

Suicidal thoughts (technically referred to as "ideations") are images, fantasies, and internal dialogue involving impulses to take one's own life. These are psychological processes with an obsessive focus on feelings of overwhelm, hopelessness, and despair.

Nearly one million people worldwide take their lives each year.

Treating suicidal patients requires immediate intervention. Psychiatric medications may help in the long term. But suicidal impulses are urgent.

IV ketamine treatments are promising for treating potentially fatal impulses within hours, not months. Studies suggesting ketamine may effectively treat suicidal ideations in emergencies are not new. Unfortunately, few patients contemplating suicide are offered this option.

Rigorous studies of ketamine's impact on suicidal ideations are limited and use small populations. Witnesses to the anti-suicidal effect are often clinicians and families of patients who observe this "superpower" firsthand. For them, seeing is believing: ketamine saves lives.

Along with that most precious outcome, it can also retrieve patients from desperate moods, decreasing symptoms of anger, aggression, irritability, and helplessness. This might be accomplished without the one to three-month delay characteristic of other medications.

Post-Traumatic Stress Disorder

PTSD is a prolonged psychological state of injury pursuant to a traumatic event. Such events generally involve violence (such as combat or sexual assault), serious injury (from accidents), and severe acute or chronic periods of high stress (scarcity of money and other resources, high-stakes employment, or academic pursuit). Recurrent, distressing memories, flashbacks, and nightmares are common symptoms.

Worldwide statistics suggest PTSD impacts approximately 4 percent of the population. In the U.S., war veterans suffer disproportionately, creating a large pool of disabled soldiers (estimated at one-fourth of the veteran population). Thankfully, this condition is better recognized and more successfully treated than before.

Many studies have shown that ketamine is effective at reducing PTSD symptoms. While temporary, even one intravenous treatment session frequently provides relief. Studies also show ketamine as superior to psychotherapy alone, both in terms of the time required to curtail symptoms and the perseverance of those effects. Even patients whose condition is unresponsive to standard treatments frequently see better results.

Ketamine infusion therapy is being discussed and prescribed more often for PTSD. Mounting anecdotal and clinical evidence suggests a potentially more prominent treatment role for ketamine going forward. Some patients report relief after only one infusion.

Bipolar Disorder

Bipolar disorder is a mental health condition characterized by extreme mood swings, manic episodes, and prolonged depression. The World Health Organization reports it as the sixth-leading cause of disability worldwide. Among the variety of mental health patients, bipolar sufferers are the most likely to commit suicide. This condition is frequently more treatment-resistant than standard depression.

We need new therapies for bipolar disorder. Ketamine's antidepressant and anti-suicidal properties make it a strong candidate for a role in this condition's management.

Most available ketamine (and esketamine) studies focus on conventional depression. However, researchers are seeing ketamine as a helpful adjuvant in treating bipolar disorder in both the short- and long-term. Whether administered intravenously or sublingually, ketamine is shown to reduce symptoms and improve mood in a matter of hours to days. It also works when combined with other psychiatric medications.

Ketamine therapy offers additional, compelling advantages. Treating bipolar disorder with ketamine is less invasive than other treatments, such as electroconvulsive therapy and deep brain stimulation. Administering ketamine by IV does not require an anesthesiologist on-site, permitting its use in outpatient clinics. It is generally considered safe and tolerable for those diagnosed with bipolar disorder.

Obsessive-Compulsive Disorder

Obsessions are distressing, anxiety-provoking, intrusive, repetitive, and persistent thoughts and feelings. Compulsions are hard-to-resist behaviors that attempt to alleviate the psychological and emotional stress created by the obsessions. OCD is characterized by the continual cycles between obsessions and compulsions. Approximately 1 in 50 people worldwide have OCD.

Roughly one in three individuals with OCD do not report significant benefits from standard therapies like cognitive behavioral therapy or antidepressants.

Furthermore, it takes about two to three months to see therapeutic effects, even when they're ultimately helpful. Antidepressants take longer to work for OCD and require higher doses than when used for depression. Treatment's failure to provide symptomatic relief is a source of decreased quality of life for many of these patients.

Ketamine benefits from a fast onset and is generally well-tolerated. A 2021 review of previous studies evaluated ketamine's therapeutic potential for managing OCD. Researchers noted that ketamine infusions lessened OCD symptoms rapidly and with effects lasting for days to weeks.

Anxiety

Everyone experiences fearful thoughts and worries. However, clinical anxiety is diagnosed when related symptoms become overwhelming or affect one's ability to function. Severe, acute anxiety episodes like panic attacks and chronic, high-stress levels can keep patients from doing things they love, staying productive, and carrying out basic activities. Intense anxiety wears on the body and the mind, often resulting in depression. Estimates put the worldwide rate of anxiety disorders at 4 percent.

While being applied to other situations, physicians have noted ketamine's secondary effect of soothing anxiety. Low-dose IV ketamine infusions are best known for treating depression, but they may also help with anxiety disorders.

A 2017 study looked at the effect of ketamine treatment on patients with generalized anxiety disorder and social anxiety disorder who were not currently depressed but also not responding to standard anti-anxiety medications. The study concluded that ketamine was safe, well-tolerated, and had potential as an anti-anxiety medication.

Chronic or severe pain

Pain is the experience of psychological, emotional, and physical discomfort. The problem of difficult-to-treat chronic pain is a worldwide challenge, begging for resolution. An estimated 20% of the world's population suffers from a pain condition. Ketamine is joining the collection of desperately needed options for this patient group.

Years of research and clinical practice continue to reveal the dangers and failures of limiting the treatment of chronic pain to opioid, anti-epileptic, and antidepressant drugs. Most concerning are opioids due to their highly addictive nature. Patients on this class of drugs frequently become tolerant and require higher doses to maintain relief. Consequently, this nation is caught in an opioid epidemic with high social and economic costs, including the loss of life on a large scale. One of ketamine's attractive properties is not being an opioid.

Anecdotal evidence suggests that over 50 percent of ketamine infusion patients report significant relief, with 7 out of 10 citing varying degrees of functional recovery proceeding therapy.

Chronic pain may decrease during or after an infusion or require successive treatments. Some patients enjoy prolonged relief, especially from neuropathy.

Pain patients frequently experience depressive symptoms, drowsiness, dizziness, or memory impairment. Because ketamine can improve mood, employing ketamine in these cases may offer a double benefit.

Ketamine infusions for pain may also have a breakthrough and prolonged analgesic effect on conditions resistant to other treatments. One example of this is a complex regional pain syndrome, a severe chronic pain condition that can arise after bodily injury, surgery, a stroke, or a heart attack. However, the long-term impact of high-dose ketamine treatment for pain is unknown and concerning.

The good news is that IV ketamine therapy may be helpful in a broad spectrum of pain conditions: migraine, neuropathy, fibromyalgia, spinal cord injury, limb ischemia pain, phantom limb pain, whiplash, and temporomandibular joint pain.

Migraines

Migraines are recurring headaches that often occur along with nausea and other symptoms. They are among the most common neurological diseases worldwide, with an estimated 1.1 billion sufferers globally as of 2019. Migraines, tension-type headaches, and medication-overuse headaches are some of the most common disorders associated with disability and ill health.

Ketamine has been researched as an abortive therapy (relief for in-progress migraines) since 1995. Multiple studies have demonstrated its ability to alleviate attacks and reduce pain intensity, though results are mixed. More studies are needed to better understand appropriate dosing and its correspondence to safety and efficacy.

Neuropathy

Neuropathy, or nerve pain, is a challenging pain disorder involving damage to the nervous system, a vast communication network broadcasting signals throughout the brain, spinal cord, and the rest of the body. Approximately one in thirty people worldwide suffer from this condition. Neuropathic pain exerts multiple harmful effects on patients–negatively affecting careers and relationships, endangering their physical safety, and limiting daily function.

Ketamine inhibits pain receptor activity in the nervous system, providing relief (even for opioid-tolerant patients). Having a well-tolerated side effect profile relative to opioids and other pain relievers highlights its therapeutic potential. Compared to the protocols for psychiatric conditions, higher ketamine doses, with more frequent treatments of longer length, provide greater relief of symptoms.

One key question is how to use ketamine for severe pain relief over the long term without causing injury or dependence. These are serious concerns for patients with chronic neuropathic disorders requiring frequent and high-dose treatment. Most medical applications of ketamine to pain have been short-term, making these treatments better understood than those given in the long term.

Addiction

Drug addiction is a chronic, relapsing brain disorder characterized by compulsive drug seeking despite adverse consequences. The causes are complex, but genetics, environment, and mental health status undeniably influence drug use and subsequent addiction. Approximately 40 million people worldwide are burdened by substance use disorders.

Substance addictions are stigmatized and treated as criminal justice issues, with users fined, imprisoned, or sent to mandatory programs. Overwhelming evidence indicates that these approaches exacerbate the problem. Redirection into therapeutic healthcare rather than incarceration is becoming recognized as a more sensible option.

There are mainstream treatments with maintenance medications such as methadone and buprenorphine for opioid addiction. Other approaches include psychotherapy, residential rehabilitation, and support groups like Alcoholics and Narcotics Anonymous. Unfortunately, addictions are frequently resistant to treatment.

A 2018 review found ketamine could help treat opioid, alcohol, and cocaine addictions. Ketamine may lessen the intensity of cravings and other withdrawal symptoms while curbing the depressive symptoms that make quitting difficult. This combination of benefits may reduce relapse rates.

Ketamine's ability to alleviate depression and PTSD is significant. These two conditions frequently fuel substance abuse as the sufferer attempts to escape their psychological and emotional pain. By countering the emotional health symptoms, ketamine may discourage addictive responses.

Addiction patients need new tools to loosen the grip of their illness. Ketamine may help. Clinics nationwide are already applying this therapy. It faces skepticism, though, because of its associations in the public consciousness with illicit use.

Dementia

Dementia is a general term for deficits in memory, problem-solving, language, and thinking abilities that are severe enough to interfere with daily life. Although it mainly affects older people, it is not a part of normal aging. It is a syndrome, usually of a progressive or chronic nature, with a deterioration in cognitive function beyond the effects of regular aging. Fifty million people have dementia worldwide, with about ten million new cases diagnosed yearly.

To appreciate the possibilities of using ketamine in the fight against dementia, we first need to examine the links between it and depression.

Depression and dementia are often comorbid conditions. In fact, depression may be a risk factor for the diagnosis of dementia. Plus, the medications for depression may increase the risk of dementia. Successfully alleviating depression may lessen the chances of experiencing cognitive impairments in later life. If nothing else, ketamine may relieve the depression dementia patients commonly endure.

One problem with ketamine therapy as applied to dementia is the impact of its psychoactive effects. Additional caution is warranted because these effects mimic symptoms we already find concerning in dementia patients. Ketamine, even when administered in sub-anesthetic doses, can elicit confusion, disrupt memory, induce hallucinations, and trigger psychotic events.

16

TRIANGULATING YOUR TREATMENTS

ARE YOU EXHAUSTED FROM COMBATING ILLNESS? COPING WITH A severe health problem takes a lot of physical and mental energy. It makes managing life's many responsibilities just that much harder.

Believe me, I can relate. I've spent a good portion of my adult life requiring assistance from loved ones in every area: medicine, insurance, finances, career decisions, and housing. And that's not all. Let's just say I am well-acquainted with feeling helpless and embarrassed by my inability to fulfill my adult responsibilities.

Side effects of the medications, many of which cause cognitive slowdown, confusion, and difficulty concentrating, compound the problem.

In the fog of physical and emotional pain, high stress, and heavy medications, you may struggle to evaluate ketamine's benefits. It is normal to wonder if and when these treatments are helping you.

How long does it take to kick in? What are the signs? Both are great questions.

I call my approach to answering them the Golden Triangle.

This is how it works: Most of us have three groups monitoring our status: our physicians, therapists and counselors, and family and friends.

Think of these three groups as points of a triangle.

You are in the middle of the triangle. When you combine your own internal experience with the feedback from the three groups surrounding you, the 360-degree reality of your health status emerges.

Your doctor tracks your treatment results. Your therapist considers your needs and teaches the appropriate coping skills. Frequently, families carry the most profound insights–not only because of their close contact but because they watch you change over time. They know your patterns. You cannot hide your life's reality from them like you can from your medical team.

You can see where this is going. Consulting the triangle's three points would reveal much if I wanted a holistic picture of your condition and progress.

This is the way I triangulate my position in treatment. If it were based solely on my judgment, I would discount the perspectives of others who see my case from the outside. Have you ever been told you seemed better or worse than you thought? I have. It's common. That's why medicine is a team sport.

So, I keep a log. Simply put, I take notes from people on the triangle's three points.

This practice provides these benefits:

1. Helps you assess whether ketamine is helping and to what degree.

2. Enables higher quality feedback to your medical team, empowering them to adjust your treatment appropriately.

3. Provides you with a sense of control over what's happening and what to do next.

This book's free bonus materials include my version of this log. Please see *findketamine.com/bookvideos*

Tips:

Keep your ketamine physician apprised of your triangle's feedback. The more feedback you give, the more everyone can help you. If you ever receive confusing or concerning feedback, share it with the other two groups in your triangle.

The Golden Triangle helps inform your treatment plan and helps track your cumulative gains.

Many clinicians and patients believe that ketamine's rejuvenation of the brain does not end after an infusion but accumulates over successive treatments. While the ketamine metabolites do not remain in your system for long, I've observed a continuity of positive cumulative effects in myself and others. This is especially true when you combine your treatment regimen with psychotherapy and take action on your discoveries.

One concrete example of this incremental growth relates to memory. After decades of medications and a bout of encephalitis, my brain is certainly not in top shape. Even to this day, my daily functionality related to short-term memory is limited. Having said that, since I began ketamine treatments four years ago, my long-term memory has improved significantly.

At first, it was subtle. I'd be discussing a family memory, and details about who said what and why all became clearer. Without any prior map of what I remembered or not, I just assumed that my recollections emerged from the pool of memories we all can typically access.

Only when others pointed out the improvement in my memory did I start paying more attention. Sure enough, regarding the long term, I began noticing more transparent windows into memorable happenings.

For instance, take my sister's Barbie dolls that I would mangle after coming home from elementary school. I can see those poor plastic mannequins as clearly as the day I destroyed them. And that alleyway behind my childhood home that hosted the perennial blackberry tree? I could draw the whole trunk for you.

There are endless examples. And I know they are significant because I clearly remember how all these ancient memories were so recently absent.

17

SAFETY AND SIDE EFFECTS

KETAMINE IS NOT FREE FROM SIDE EFFECTS. ITS SAFE USE REQUIRES professional consideration and supervision. Its adverse effects depend on several factors, including which other medications are in the mix.

Most ketamine patients have been or still are on other medications. Because their prescriptions are not working or have unbearable side effects is precisely why they are seeking ketamine treatment.

Potential patients often ask if they can undergo low-dose IV ketamine infusions while on other prescription medications. In many cases, the answer is yes. However, the physician will review each patient's medication regimen.

Contraindications include certain drugs and supplements. Some substances require a "wash out" period, as they must completely evacuate the body. Specifying a certain period of abstinence from medications may also be an option.

In my case, my doctor suggested I remain on my current medication regimen, with some temporary modifications around the treatment day.

My doctor instructed me to refrain from taking Klonopin and Lamictal, both psychiatric medications, for twelve hours before my IV ketamine infusion.

Usually prescribed for anxiety, Klonopin is a benzodiazepine. Other drugs in this category include Valium, Xanax, and Ativan.

Benzodiazepines may interfere by lessening the therapeutic value of ketamine treatments, altering the ketamine "experience," and presenting unexpected interactions.

Being off of "benzos" and going into ketamine treatment may be ideal. Some doctors even recommend several weeks of discontinued benzodiazepine use before IV ketamine treatments.

The problem is that many patients have a long history of legal benzodiazepine use, are currently on a benzodiazepine, and cannot discontinue them due to severe withdrawal symptoms, which can be fatal.

In my case, I am still receiving ketamine benefits despite legally prescribed, long-term benzodiazepine use. This is because my doctor instructed me on the window of time I need to hold off on my benzodiazepine medication before each infusion.

There is still much we don't know. The benzodiazepine dosage, length of use, and other factors may be important. Perhaps because I use a small dose of Klonopin, the twelve-hour window before my ketamine treatment is enough to allow effective treatment. Again, fully disclose your regimen to your physician and follow their instructions.

Lamictal is often used to treat bipolar depression. When it works, it is a useful antidepressant unlikely to trigger mania. However, it may inhibit ketamine's therapeutic effects. Or it may trigger positive, synergistic action. Studies have yet to settle this matter conclusively.

Do not make this decision alone. Only your doctor can analyze your case specifically. Don't forget to disclose nutritional supplementations and recreational drugs, as any potential interaction could be severe.

Ketamine may interact with a variety of drugs, including ADHD medications such as Adderall, certain antidepressant drugs, and central nervous system depressants like alcohol, opiates, allergy medicine, rifampin, and ticlopidine.

Technically, ketamine poses interaction risks with a raft of medications in addition to those above. However, at least anecdotally speaking, I rarely hear of patients unable to participate in ketamine therapy due to their medication regimens. This is great news because many people needing ketamine treatments are already on prescriptions and supplements.

I'm usually on five to six medications: mood stabilizers, antidepressants, benzodiazepines, beta-blockers, and antihistamines. These medications address my comorbid diagnoses of depression, bipolar disorder, and OCD. When treating several conditions, it's common to depend on various medications, some to manage your symptoms and others to manage the side effects of medicating those symptoms. It can be complicated and exhausting. Thankfully, there are usually ways to still receive ketamine therapy.

In 2015, a study focused on the safety, tolerability, and acceptability of ketamine in treatment-resistant depression observed that only 1.9 percent of infusions were discontinued due to side effects. In the first four hours after the infusion, the most common adverse reactions reported were drowsiness, dizziness, poor coordination, blurred vision, and feeling strange or unreal. Ketamine use was associated with small but significant increases in psychotic and dissociative symptoms. The researchers in this study concluded that ketamine was safe and well-tolerated.

However, there are exceptional cases. Here is a partial list of those for whom ketamine may be inadvisable.

- Patients with underlying conditions in which increased blood pressure could increase the risk of cardiovascular complications like angina, heart failure, aortic dissection, uncontrolled hypertension, or aneurysms.

- People with severe head injuries, glaucoma, and hyperthyroidism.

- Patients hypersensitive to ketamine or carrying a diagnosis of schizophrenia or bipolar condition.

- Women who are pregnant or breastfeeding.

- Patients with a history of addiction.

18

JUGGLING MEDICATIONS

FINDING THE RIGHT COMBINATIONS OF MEDICATIONS FOR MANAGING complex medical conditions is challenging. As someone on many medications, I frequently have to adjust them to strengthen their therapeutic effects or dial down their unwanted side effects. Juggling these tradeoffs is an art and a science, requiring a guiding philosophy.

The science: One advantage of living in this age of psychiatric therapy is the institutional knowledge of what medication to give to whom, when, and in what dose. Intervening in many diseases is moderately formulaic and represented in treatment algorithms–flow charts of recommended decisions in a patient's chronology of care. The "standard of care" is represented in these charts.

These decision trees guide physicians on best practices. For instance, when someone shows depressive symptoms, treatment guidelines may first recommend an antidepressant. If that doesn't work, the algorithm may suggest other antidepressants from different classes. If the chart's recommendations have yet to gain traction, the next step may be adding an antipsychotic.

The upside of the flowchart approach is that many years of experience by many practitioners are condensed into *if-then* rules–simple, step-by-step paths to reasonably good results. The downside is that not everyone responds to these same steps. For instance, antidepressants don't work for everyone. And, even as one continues down the suggested path of trying this and that, there's still no guarantee of a better outcome.

People well-served by the algorithm are delighted. They've potentially skipped years of agony. But what if this treatment path isn't working for you? What if you're on your fifth antidepressant and you're still depressed? Suddenly, relying on a failed lockstep approach doesn't sound so good. Maybe the next recommended step won't work, either. Or the next. Or the next.

The art: For those not finding relief from following the "playbook," its existence isn't comforting. It may even impede treatment. When a physician is married to the playbook, which they could be as a matter of following the standard of care or because they've seen it work, we may have trouble finding a second opinion on an alternate treatment path. This happened to me repeatedly as I tried dozens of medications in the twenty-five years before I found ketamine. It's not that my doctors were all incompetent. I just was not improving through the standard treatment regimen. This is where the "art" of doctoring comes in. Just because there's a commonly followed standard of care for your condition, your physician still has leeway to customize your options.

For instance, psychiatrists often observe over time that particular medications work better than others for people with specific diagnoses. An abundance of clinical data may not bear out their conclusions. They may not be able to objectively prove the benefit of this optional treatment approach. But, by virtue of their education, experience, and intuition, their approach may lead to exceptional outcomes.

Sometimes, the benefit of getting a second opinion comes from this artistic, experiential, and intuitive side that varies among physicians.

The philosophy: As patients, we all bring a philosophy to our medical situation. For instance, some people promptly discover an effective medication and leave it at that. They're not trying to optimize it or find something more powerful but with fewer side effects (which may or may not exist). They don't shop for doctors and treatments. They're happy with moderate relief and stick it out.

Other people, including me, cannot function without excellent treatment. I simply can't do with a "little" relief. Nor can some of the side effects of my medications merely be ignored. Therefore, my philosophy is patience with the long journey toward better days. It means consulting with multiple doctors, trying many treatments, and enduring the cycles of hope and despair. I'm just glad that ketamine is pretty tolerant of my medication changes.

But it still leaves the question of how my provider and I are supposed to intelligently adjust my ketamine treatments amid these alterations in my drug regimen. If I'm on fewer medications, for instance, and I have a ketamine session coming up, does that mean we should increase or decrease my ketamine dose?

During the past four years that I've received ketamine infusions, I've shown up at the clinic on more or fewer medications and in better or worse condition. Before each ketamine procedure, the staff 1) administers a paper-based questionnaire for feedback on my depression and anxiety symptoms, 2) asks me to orally report on how the last treatment went, and 3) inquires about how I have felt since. These logs track my reaction to treatment and inform the plan as we advance.

19

KETAMINE AIN'T CHEAP

Low-dose intravenous infusions of ketamine are expensive, mainly because obtaining insurance reimbursement can be difficult.

Treatments range from approximately $300 to $800 per session. Five to six sessions are considered an initial treatment plan— enough to give insight into ketamine's expected impact on your symptoms and whether continuing the treatment makes sense.

Chronic pain conditions, though, frequently require much longer sessions and costs that can exceed $1,000 per therapy.

Ketamine itself is not under patent and is very inexpensive. High treatment costs come from the infrastructure of running a clinic with leasing space, liability insurance, staff, equipment, and more.

Some ketamine clinics provide savings through package deals or membership plans. Others offer sliding scale or income-based pricing. Each clinic has its policies for treatment consultations.

Esketamine nasal treatments also cost several hundred dollars. However, when prescribed for treatment-resistant depression or suicidal thoughts, they may be covered by insurance or subsidized by the drug's manufacturer, Janssen Pharmaceuticals.

Another alternative to intravenous ketamine is at-home ketamine therapy with rapid dissolving tablets. The price of this approach varies considerably and prevents a direct comparison between providers. Some services only offer prescriptions. Others mandate ongoing psychotherapy and multiple telehealth appointments with prescribers. Here is my candid, personal opinion after trying this form of therapy:

FindKetamine.com/bookvideos

In summary, unless you are enrolled in a clinical trial or your insurance is paying, ketamine therapy can be hard to afford.

20

HOW TO AFFORD TREATMENT

MEDICAL BILLS ARE THE NUMBER ONE CAUSE OF BANKRUPTCY IN THE U.S. With medical treatments that can run into millions of dollars, even people with excellent employer-backed insurance can amass bills that exceed virtually anyone's savings.

Despite my hard work, this happened to me:

I was a year out of university with a well-paying job. Plus, I was investing in real estate with my mom.

After a year and a half, my health went downhill. The stress at work amplified my depression and OCD. More meds were piled on. Not only did I not feel better, but the side effects intensified.

In my job, I traveled every week. Exhaustion from that, combined with the medications, made me extra tired. My mind was racing as my body weakened. All of this turned me into a zombie. I'd show up hours late for work. I simply couldn't wake up.

Before long, I lost all concentration. Sadness and fear took over. These emotions triggered outright panic. Going on disability leave was my only option. Little did I know that I would remain in this state for more than a year.

My house became my hospital and my prison. I locked myself away. Human Resources sent me disability paperwork. My mom had to fill it out.

With my income at a standstill and more than a year of medical bills, I had to declare bankruptcy. I lost my investment properties, my good credit, and my dignity.

Sitting in the attorney's office for the bankruptcy procedure, I was mortified. Even though I was a legitimate mess, I was afraid he wouldn't believe me; he'd see a "healthy young man" and doubt the seriousness of my situation.

Mercifully, he was a great guy and eventually became a friend. Regardless, I still lost everything.

Because I've been through the process of recovering from massive debt and abysmal credit ratings, I've learned a bit about the process. The most important thing for you to know is that you certainly can fight your way back, but it will take time, education, and guidance.

No matter your financial situation, you deserve the best health-care possible. Sometimes, that means a long and frustrating search for help. The answer is often just a call away from a relative or close friend. Maybe an inquiry at your place of worship? Or a community center?

But what if none of these efforts help? What if you desperately need treatment, but insurance won't cover it, and you have no one to call upon?

You can't work. You can't bring in income. You can't afford the treatments you need. So, you remain unable to work, unable to earn income, and unable to afford medical treatment. And around and around. This can be a death spiral. Nothing's sadder than losing a health battle to money.

I've been there. For my twenty-five-plus-year health journey, it's taken many friends, family, insurance consultants, research, and phone calls for me to make it to this point in my life.

But DON'T GIVE UP. I truly believe where there is a will, there's a way!

When you decide to take action and keep knocking on doors, it's hard to keep you locked out forever.

There is a plethora of payment options and ways to raise funds. They include:

Insurance reimbursement. Even though ketamine has a long history of medical use as an anesthetic, it is only now gaining attention and approval for other applications. Therefore, it can be challenging to get it covered by insurance. Treatment-resistant depression is one growing exception that some insurance companies are beginning to acknowledge.

This is the most cost-effective way to afford ketamine. With insurance footing the bill, a $500 treatment may shrink to a $20 co-pay.

Still, many insurers consider ketamine treatment "experimental" and decline coverage for that reason. Even if they agree to some reimbursement, securing it will require a lot of work. Further, the copay or deductible may exceed one's budget even with substantial reimbursement.

One exception to this is the esketamine/Spravato intranasal treatment. The FDA approved this form of ketamine therapy in 2019. Insurance frequently covers it. However, there are two issues:

- There is a debate about whether esketamine is as effective as IV ketamine.

- Even with insurance reimbursement, copays for esketamine treatment can still exceed affordability.

Some clinics assist in submitting insurance claims. All clinics should provide a "Superbill," a list of your diagnoses and the treatments you've paid for. You will need this to send to your insurance company.

Tips for winning reimbursement:

- Employ the correct CD10 codes while documenting all conditions and symptoms thoroughly.

- Follow the reimbursement protocol exactly.

- Understand that processing your claim may take weeks or months. Don't give up.

- Check in with your insurance company regularly. Ask for the status. If your claim is rejected, request instructions for the appeal process.

- Know that insurers may cover differing percentages governed by which providers are within their network, your coverage tier, deductibles, and other factors.

- If you run into an insurer that refuses to reimburse you, citing ketamine as "experimental," use doctor's notes, your prior medical record, and the clinical studies referenced in the "endnotes" portion of this book to prove your case.

Government programs. Aid comes in many forms in many circumstances. Some programs provide funds directly for care. Others make health insurance more affordable. Still others are geared toward helping particular populations, such as veterans.

Each government fund has different eligibility requirements. You may need to be a state resident, under a certain age, below a certain income, or with a specific diagnosis. Other possible criteria may be your current insurance coverage, income, family size, assets, military service, and employment status.

Tons of these programs exist; you must sift through them, visit their websites, and make phone calls. If you are unable to do it, ask a friend or a caregiver. If not them, try a social worker or patient advocate.

As much as I'd like to guarantee that one of these programs will solve your payment challenges, I can't. Instead, I have compiled a list of aid programs within your free *bonus materials*.

Crowdfunding. Medical journeys are emotional and can be both inspiring and tragic. Whether in our own lives or the lives of loved ones, we have all witnessed the ravages of health problems. For this reason, many people relate to medical needs and would like to help.

Medical crowdfunding raises money online for medical expenses. Perhaps you've even participated in it. This approach is growing in popularity due to the ease of the technology behind it.

Anyone can donate to a crowdfunding effort. It often begins within one's network of family, friends, colleagues, and community. You will see these campaigns on social platforms like Facebook, where fundraisers efficiently get the word out.

Most of us are not professional fundraisers. We are probably not the best at putting together the materials that tell the story of need and persuade people to pitch in.

Some fundraising platforms offer templates for creating a solid proposal for potential donors. These help you articulate what you need, why, and when. Using these outlines, you'll avoid errors and make a professional effort.

Raising funds for medical procedures used to be slow, difficult to scale, and hampered by geographical location. Today, social networking technology can publish a campaign in minutes, instantly reaching an unlimited number of people anywhere in the world.

Before the explosion of the Internet, fundraisers required manual collections of checks and cash—a time-intensive effort fraught with security risks.

Medical crowdfunding sites have built-in payment systems that make collecting gifts for your fundraiser fast, secure, and easy.

Fundraising fraud creates skeptics among potential donors and hurts everyone who legitimately needs help. Legitimate fundraising platforms require payout verification and employ both automatic and human-based fraud detection strategies. If a platform loses its good reputation for hosting and executing worthwhile campaigns, its future suffers. Its operators need to scrutinize each campaign that runs on their platform.

Despite its advantages, crowdfunding still requires time and energy. Setting up a campaign online and kicking back to wait for donations is not enough.

You still have to gather the particulars, take photos, and create postings to spread the word.

Crowdfunding services are plentiful. Sites like cofundhealth.com and peoplepledge.org can power your fundraising campaign. GoFundMe.com is perhaps the best-known crowdfunding site. It is generally regarded as trusted, reliable, and worth the small fee. Donors are asked to help defray the costs, too.

Friends and family. Most of us have a hard time asking for help. It can be difficult even if we need it and are fortunate enough to have people who care about us. We may fear rejection or feel we are asking too much. Ironically, we're often glad to help when other people ask. But we tend to remain quiet when it's the other way around.

But when we are dealing with a serious illness and can't afford the treatment we need, it can force us to reach out to others.

In doing so, and to preserve these precious relationships, it's essential to address these questions:

- Why are you asking?
- Is it a severe problem?
- Are you in immediate need?
- What happens if you get help with treatment?
- What happens if you don't?

Helping people understand the importance of their assistance can go a long way. Educating them about your situation will make them more sympathetic to your cause, even if they haven't been in your shoes.

Sometimes, we need help from people with whom we are not on the best terms. It could be a small rift or a long-standing wound.

Asking for forgiveness and mending relationships is always healthy for the body and the mind. But in dire circumstances, it can become a necessity.

Maybe you feel the bad blood was not your fault; perhaps you don't even know what spawned it. Either way, it's hard for someone to come to your aid while that barrier remains. Asking for forgiveness can be difficult and awkward, especially if you're not used to doing so.

You may be surprised how far a sincere apology can go; maybe the person you're thinking about approaching was already feeling bad about the wedge between you. Returning to good terms can restore the mutual commitment to assisting one another in tough times.

Experts. You may have trouble explaining your condition. To do so, provide an evidence-backed reason for your request.

People frequently want to help but don't fully understand the situation. Make them more comfortable by detailing the official diagnosis and treatment plan. Help them understand how their support directly increases your chances of winning this fight.

Advocates. If it's hard to ask for help or you're in a damaged relationship, advocates can help. A family member or friend may be able to reach out to people you can't approach. Additionally, hearing about someone's needs from a third party can bring credibility and induce more sympathy. Having an honest, well-respected friend approach others on your behalf can be very effective.

Rarely are fundraisers run by the person requiring help. Loved ones and friends generally publicize the cause. Similarly, charities employ spokespeople to champion their causes.

Credit. If other approaches do not work, you may need to consider credit-based options to afford treatment. These include credit cards. They are not the ideal solution, but they could be necessary.

Credit cards and various loan types each have their pros and cons. One benefit of credit products is that approval is often prompt, with the funds available in hours. Speed is a factor when someone is suffering and potentially suicidal.

One downside is that inexpensive credit is often available only to those who "don't need it" because they already have an excellent credit rating and a high income. Further, when credit is available to people without these prerequisites, it is usually more expensive and carries higher penalties for default. The good news is that credit cards are available for virtually every credit score.

Installment and personal loans. Called by many names, loans and credit lines may fit your needs. With loans, you borrow an amount of money for a specific term. You repay that loan with interest and other fees. Credit lines allow you to borrow up to a maximum amount, repay that (in full or in part), and draw upon it again up to that maximum amount. Both of these may help you pay for treatment when money is tight.

I hope that one day soon, everyone who needs ketamine treatments can easily afford them.

21

FREQUENTLY ASKED QUESTIONS

THE POTENTIAL BENEFITS OF KETAMINE FOR MENTAL HEALTH conditions are attracting attention. Here is a comprehensive list of questions and answers about its use:

Q. Is ketamine used for mental health challenges?

A. Currently, ketamine is prescribed for treatment-resistant depression, PTSD, bipolar disorder, obsessive-compulsive disorder, suicidal thoughts, and anxiety.

Whether it will work in your particular case cannot be guaranteed.

Ketamine's targeted use for psychiatric disorders is still in its early stages. However, studies are proliferating and yielding positive results.

Q. Is ketamine used to treat pain?

A. Ketamine is useful as an anesthetic partly because of its pain-relieving properties. Now, it is receiving particular interest as a much-needed alternative to opioids.

Currently, ketamine is prescribed for chronic regional pain syndrome, migraines, neuropathy, and other pain disorders.

Q. Is ketamine used to treat addiction?

There is evidence of ketamine assisting in the breaking of addiction. This includes substance abuse and behavioral addictions. Some clinics specialize in treating addiction through this branch of ketamine therapy.

Q. What are ketamine's side effects?

A. The most common effects are dissociation, increased pulse and blood pressure, dizziness, blurry vision, headache, nausea, poor coordination, and restlessness. However, nausea and dizziness are usually prevented by medication administered before your session.

Anyone receiving ketamine should not drive, use heavy machinery, or participate in any dangerous activity for up to twenty-four hours after treatment for these reasons.

Allergic reactions can range from mild itchiness to life-threatening anaphylaxis. The spectrum includes breathing difficulties, hives, and swelling of the face, lips, throat, and tongue.

Cardiovascular symptoms: abnormal heart rhythm, higher blood pressure, left ventricular dysfunction in individuals with heart failure, and severe events such as respiratory and cardiac arrest.

Gastrointestinal symptoms: lack of appetite, nausea, and vomiting.

Musculoskeletal symptoms: muscle stiffness, seizure-like symptoms, and increased muscular tone.

Neurologic: confusion, seizures, dizziness, drowsiness, and vertigo.

Eyes: double vision, increased intraocular pressure, and nystagmus.

Psychiatric symptoms: amnesia, anxiety, confusion, depression, disorientation, dysphoria, dissociative state, emergence phenomena/delirium, hallucinations, flashbacks, unusual thoughts, extreme fear, excitement, irrational behavior, and insomnia.

Respiratory: apnea, increased laryngeal and tracheal secretions, laryngospasm, and respiratory depression.

Skin symptoms are rarely documented but may include swelling and pain at the injection site.

Even with over fifty treatments under my belt, I have experienced only a handful of minor effects that dissipated immediately after the therapy session.

Q. Is it safe to use ketamine recreationally?

A. No. When used recreationally, risks include tolerance, dependence, and addiction. If abruptly discontinued, withdrawal symptoms may occur. Unguided and unmonitored administration of ketamine can be addictive and fatal.

Q. Is long-term ketamine therapy dangerous?

A. Prolonged use of ketamine may affect the body. It is metabolized in the liver and excreted through the kidneys. High doses (usually much higher than those used in the IV ketamine treatments we've been discussing) can damage these vital organs. Chronic, high-dose intake can also injure the bladder.

Q. Is ketamine prescribed alongside other medications?

A. One stand-out benefit versus other psychiatric medications is the seeming absence of the complications of other augmenting agents such as antipsychotics, which can cause significant, irreversible injuries such as tardive dyskinesia (involuntary movements of the face and jaw) or metabolic disorders like diabetes.

Q. Does ketamine cause hallucinations?

A. This class of drug can cause hallucinations at high doses. Comorbid illness may impact the likelihood or degree of this effect.

Q. Does ketamine trigger mania in bipolar patients?

A. This is a common question that results from ketamine's strong anti-depressant effects. The safety of using ketamine to treat a bipolar diagnosis requires discussion with your physician. However, as someone with bipolar disorder, I have not experienced this issue during treatment.

Q. Isn't ketamine a club drug or an animal tranquilizer?

A. Ketamine has a reputation outside of the medical community as a "club drug," sometimes called Special K. Meanwhile, the World Health Organization lists ketamine as an essential medicine. Without its availability for anesthesia and pain relief, millions would suffer and die unnecessarily. That said, some people seek out ketamine illegally and abuse it recreationally.

Referring to this invaluable medicine as an "animal tranquilizer" is misguided as well. For one, veterinarians use ketamine for anesthesia and pain relief, just as your physician does. Two, there is nothing out of place about pharmaceuticals with multiple uses, even among mammals.

Q. Is ketamine safe?

A. Ketamine benefits from a long history of use as a safe and effective pharmaceutical agent. The last decade birthed an explosion of interest in psychedelic and dissociative therapies. Medical interventions affecting consciousness are always mysterious, creating promise and paranoia. Don't prejudge; talk with your physician.

Q. Is ketamine addictive?

A. Ketamine, like any drug, is susceptible to abuse. Its popularity in the underground dance scene, known as "Special K," nearly ruined the open-minded attitude seen today in the medical community.

"Outside of the clinic, ketamine can cause tragedies, but in the right hands, it is a miracle," noted John Abenstein, president of the American Society of Anesthesiologists.

Recreational ketamine abuse can injure the cardiovascular, cognitive, respiratory, reproductive, and immune systems.

Prescribed and supervised low-dose applications make abuse difficult.

As with most drug abuse, the initial experiences may produce relaxation or euphoria. However, when taken too frequently or in excessive amounts, k-holes and the inability to interact safely with one's surroundings may result. That's why IV ketamine therapy is given in a controlled medical environment by trained staff.

For the recreational user, breaking an addiction to ketamine may not be easy. Cravings, shakes, tremors, hallucinations, heavy sweating, and other dramatic reactions similar to heroin withdrawal can plague recreational abusers.

For all these reasons, the patient's history of addiction factors into the decision behind ketamine's prescription. Patients with extant or prior addictions may not be good candidates.

As the body of ketamine treatment experience grows, our understanding of safe, effective protocols that minimize the chances of dependency will likewise expand.

Q. What are the side effects of esketamine/Spravato?

A. Side effects associated with esketamine use are dissociation, distortion of time and space, dizziness, nausea, sedation, vertigo, headache, dysgeusia (altered perception of taste), hypoesthesia (decreased awareness of sensory input), anxiety, lethargy, high blood pressure, increased heart rate, digestive symptoms, insomnia, feeling intoxicated, speech impairment, euphoric mood, excessive sweating, mental impairment, tremor, and frequent urination.

Q. What are esketamine's contraindications?

A. Esketamine is contraindicated in individuals with increased blood pressure or intracranial pressure that may lead to severe cardiovascular side effects. Intracerebral bleeding and hypersensitivity to esketamine, ketamine, or other ingredients from the drug are also contraindications.

Because it is applied through a nasal inhaler, such side effects as nasal discomfort, throat irritation, and dry mouth may occur.

Like ketamine, esketamine may impair your ability to drive a motor vehicle or operate machinery. Those who take the drug should not engage in activities requiring mental alertness and motor coordination.

Esketamine should not be used during pregnancy or lactation.

Doctor referrals

Q. Do I need to be referred by my doctor to receive ketamine infusions?

A. State regulations and insurance guidelines may vary. Coordination with your broader medical team is recommended.

Q. Who should the referral come from?

A. If a referral is necessary, it generally comes from the physician treating the condition for which you seek ketamine.

Q. What if I don't have a doctor?

A. Any licensed physician can prescribe ketamine. Frequently, a medical consultation at a ketamine clinic is sufficient to begin treatment.

Adjunct care

Q. What are ketamine-assisted therapy and ketamine-assisted psychotherapy?

A. Often used interchangeably, these psychological approaches employ professional therapists to work with patients before, during, and after their ketamine treatment. Ketamine's dissociative properties can enhance the effectiveness of these talk therapies.

Q. Should I combine ketamine with psychological therapy?

A. There is evidence that combining therapy with ketamine treatment yields better results than ketamine alone.

Q. Will I have access to this additional treatment?

A. Some clinics have an on-site specialist. Remote therapy is also available.

Q. Should I continue seeing my psychiatrist, primary care physician, or other medical team members?

A. Never make changes to your medical regimen without consulting your treating physician.

Q. Are there ketamine therapy support groups?

A. Online forums for every condition and procedure are easy to find. For instance, my Facebook group, FindKetamine, fields all questions about ketamine therapy. Tears Kuykendahl's Facebook group, KetamineAndMigraine, concentrates on ketamine therapy for migraines.

Select your ketamine clinic

Q. How do I choose a ketamine clinic for treatment?

A. Finding a ketamine clinic is not just a matter of location. It requires satisfactory answers to the right questions regarding the clinic's expertise, experience, and safety practices.

Here is a list of valuable questions:

- Am I a good candidate for treatment?

- How do we define "success" in a case like mine?

- What are my chances of success?

- Can I discontinue treatment at any time?

- Do you offer ketamine-assisted psychotherapy?

- What are the possible complications? How common are they?

- What safety measures are in place if something goes wrong?

- Are ketamine infusions safe with my other medications?

- What is the treatment schedule?

- How many treatments will I need?

- What should I tell/ask the other doctors on my medical team?

- Who provides the ketamine prescription?

- Who approves my treatment?

Q. What will the ketamine doctor ask me?

A. All of the inquiries below are appropriate:

- With what conditions do you need help?

- What is your status and prognosis?

- What medications and procedures have you tried?

- What has worked or not worked in the past?

- What are your expectations for ketamine treatment?

- Do you, or have you had, substance abuse problems?

- Is there anything about this treatment that concerns you?

Q. Are ketamine clinics safe?

A. There is no blanket answer covering every clinic. It is best to evaluate each clinic individually.

Standard regulations govern the operation of all medical clinics. However, each clinic is responsible for its compliance.

The growth of ketamine treatment centers is exploding across the U.S. and is beginning to do so in other countries. Health inspectors are likely stretched thin on time to monitor and enforce every regulation in every clinic. For this reason, you must review the credentials, ratings, and experience of each clinic's leadership.

Q. Where can I find patient reviews?

A. Some ketamine clinics post reviews and testimonials on their websites.

More objective reviews may be found on medical review sites like Vitals, *U.S. News* Doctor Rankings, and HealthGrades.

Q. Who prescribes ketamine?

A. A wide variety of clinicians have this privilege, including PCPs, psychiatrists, anesthesiologists, and more.

Q. Is there a doctor present during my infusion?

A. Medical professionals with sufficient credentials and experience should always provide and supervise your infusions. Regulations vary on what specific medical personnel must be on hand for treatment.

The main clinical director/physician is sometimes present, but not necessarily. Either way, they should have established protocols for the medical staff.

Q. How long are ketamine treatments?

A. Depending on your diagnosis's prescription, treatments may last forty minutes to several hours, with longer durations applied to pain conditions.

Your clinic will advise you on the duration of your treatment and explain the allotted time for intake and post-treatment recovery.

Treatments begin with taking vital signs and attachment to monitoring equipment for blood pressure, pulse, and oxygen saturation. The IV is inserted, and the ketamine drip begins.

Q. Can I eat or drink on the day of the procedure?

A. As ketamine is an anesthetic, eating and drinking before the procedure is prohibited. Your doctor will detail the rules.

Q. Is this an outpatient procedure?

A. Ketamine therapy is usually provided as an outpatient procedure.

Its side effects wear off quickly, usually within a few hours. Even so, patients are not permitted to drive themselves home.

Q. Why can't I drive after my infusion?

A. Ketamine's effects are intoxicating.

Q. Will someone need to accompany me?

A. Other than your driver, no accompaniment is required. However, some patients bring companions into the waiting area or the treatment room. Many people feel more comfortable having a friend or loved one along, especially during the initial sessions.

Q. Is there an age requirement to receive IV ketamine therapy?

A. There is no age limit for ketamine prescription. However, your physician may advise you to avoid ketamine at certain ages.

Q. Can ketamine be used at home?

A. Some physicians prescribe troches/lozenges as primary treatment or boosters for at-home use.

Q. Is ketamine therapy painful?

A. The IV insertion may cause a "pinch," but the treatment is not painful.

You may experience psychological or emotional distress during the dissociated aspect of your therapy. Some patients report benefits from these experiences, though they may be unpleasant at the time. Any physical or mental discomfort should be reported to your infusion staff immediately as a safety precaution.

Q. Will I be asleep during treatment?

A. Low-dose ketamine infusions do not aim to put you to sleep. However, it is common to fall asleep during treatment.

Ketamine clinic policies

Q. How quickly can I get an appointment?

A. Booking in advance is recommended. Some clinics have long wait times. However, some clinics set aside "emergency" appointment slots.

Q. Do ketamine clinics have a privacy policy?

A. Ketamine clinics must follow patient privacy laws. Before treatment, you or your legal guardian must approve any changes or releases to these rules.

Q. What are clinics' cancellation policies?

A. They vary among clinics. Policies should be disclosed on their website and by the office personnel.

Ketamine administration

Q. How is ketamine administered?

A. Ketamine is manufactured and prescribed in various forms. Each ketamine clinic may provide one or more treatment options.

Q. What are ketamine's delivery routes?

A. All of the following:

- Intravenous ketamine (IV ketamine) is used most frequently
- Intranasal ketamine (known as esketamine, brand name Spravato)
- Intramuscular or subcutaneous
- Sublingual troches
- Rectal suppositories
- Powder or crystals

Q. What is the treatment schedule?

A. Initial treatments often consist of roughly two weekly treatments for two to three weeks.

Booster and maintenance treatment schedules can vary significantly. Most patients report the need for additional sessions in weeks or months, but I occasionally hear of patients claiming no need for further treatment.

However, studies have shown that ketamine's effects on depression specifically usually tail off within two weeks. Your next steps for treatment, whether using a ketamine booster or another approach, will be addressed by your physician.

Q. Will I need ketamine treatments for the rest of my life?

Your long-term treatment plan involves staying in touch with your medical team about how you are feeling and functioning.

How often a patient may need ketamine treatments varies per patient. Receiving additional booster treatments over time is expected.

Q. Is the esketamine spray better than the IV ketamine infusions?

A. Molecularly speaking, ketamine comprises two isomers, S and K. Ketamine infusion therapy uses a combination of S and K. In contrast, esketamine intranasal spray comprises only the S. This means these two medications are not identical in every aspect.

Esketamine has been on the market for only a few years. Compared to ketamine, studies are limited regarding its efficacy and safety. Anecdotally, infusions are often considered safer and more effective.

Q. Will I be prescribed additional medication?

A. In addition to the ketamine, your physician may include small doses of medication to counteract temporary side effects such as nausea or dizziness.

Q. What should I wear to my treatment session?

A. Wear comfortable and appropriate clothing for the clinic's temperature.

Q. What should I bring with me?

A. Some patients leave everything behind, while others bring their phones and headphones for music. Sensory-dampening articles like sunglasses, eye pillows, and earplugs are recommended.

Q. What kind of music should I listen to during the infusion?

A. Music is an excellent accompaniment to ketamine treatment. Soothing instrumental music is recommended. Nature sounds are also a good option. Music with lyrics can draw attention away from the inner experience of therapy and even affect one's thoughts and feelings.

Q. Will I have privacy during my infusion?

A. Medical staff is required to check in on you periodically. You can ask for lower lighting, wear sunglasses or eye masks, and request fewer, less intrusive checks.

Q. Are clinics disability-accessible?

A. For patients requiring particular accessibility to a clinic, inquire about your needs before your office visit.

Q. Do clinics have Wi-Fi and other amenities?

A. Varies. Some ketamine clinics are simply equipped with suitable furniture and monitoring equipment. Others have Wi-Fi and even offer essential oils, massage chairs, and more.

Q. How will I feel after my ketamine infusion?

A. Some people feel rejuvenated and euphoric. Others feel the same or temporarily worse than when they arrived. Either way, the side effects of ketamine usually wear off in one to three hours.

Q. Do some clinics offer special formulations?

A. Ketamine and its combinations with other drugs are under study. Whether a proprietary formula would produce better or safer results is unknown. Combining ketamine with other medications is at your physician's discretion.

MAY I HAVE A MOMENT OF YOUR TIME?

Writing books is hard. Public vulnerability takes courage. Pulling together all of the science takes time.

Please take a moment to leave a review. I promise to read it. It makes a tremendous difference to this book's success.

Your feedback helps me improve and guides others to discover ketamine's benefits.

It's easy. You don't have to read the whole book or follow a specific formula. You can quickly select a star rating if you like. Or you can write as much as you want. Either way, you're doing me a favor.

You can leave a review at FindKetamine.com/ReviewsHelp or scan the QR code below. For both ways, once you've reached the website, you can then scroll down to click the "Write a Customer Review" button on the left side of the page.

FRANK M LIGONS

I can't thank you enough!

ACKNOWLEDGEMENTS

My sincere appreciation goes to Dr. Glen Z. Brooks, John Newmark, LPC, Terah Kuykendall, Sherry Jo Matt, Ellen D'argenzio, and the anonymous contributors.

Big hugs to my mother, Margaret, and my Aunt Beverly, who spend countless hours driving me to ketamine treatments and stopping at yummy restaurants on the way back.

Special thanks to my Aunt Diana, who always supported my journey to better health. Rest in peace.

I remain grateful to Dr. Henry Macler and his loving wife, Jean, both of whom were there for me from the very beginning of my ketamine journey.

I want to give special thanks to my Aunt Judi and my dear friend Marissa, both of whom encourage and preview my work.

Many thanks for MKF and Sticker. They're family, too.

Thankfully, I have a great medical team that cares for me. You know who you are—there are a lot of you! I won't name you for privacy's sake, but I'd like to. You each deserve a big thanks!

I have always wanted to work with an editor who I could praise in my acknowledgments for making me sound good while meeting unrealistic deadlines. Jim, thanks.

Research and Fact-checking

Brindusa Vanta, MD, DHMHS, is a medical doctor, researcher, and experienced medical writer and editor specializing in brain health. She received her MD degree from Luliu Hatieganu University of Medicine, Romania, and her HD diploma from OCHM—Canada. Doctor Vanta is a featured medical expert on Facty.com, where 25 million people seek out accurate, easy-to-understand health expertise each month.

Ermin Silajdzic, MD — Anesthesiology, Sarajevo

Kieran Doran — BMedSci (Hons) in Medical Sciences, University of Edinburgh Medical School

WJ Emalka, MBBS — National Hospital of Sri Lanka

ABOUT THE AUTHOR

Having endured decades of incapacitating anxiety and depression, Frank M. Ligons understands the burdens of chronic illness and disability. After trying dozens of medications, he finally discovered ketamine therapy. Ketamine stopped his twenty-five years of suicidal thoughts in their tracks!

He holds a Master of Science in Biomedical Informatics with co-authored research in prestigious medical journals, including the Biomedical Journal of Quality & Safety, Journal of the American Medical Directors Association, and the American Medical Informatics Association® Proceedings.

Frank has presented medical research at the National Institutes of Health, the National Library of Medicine, and the American Medical Informatics Association® Symposium.

He lives in Pittsburgh, PA, eats raw eggs, and loves his dog, Sticker.

For business inquiries, please connect at LinkedIn.com/in/frankm ligons or through info@FindKetamine.com.

SELECTED BIBLIOGRAPHY

AAN HET ROT, M., COLLINS, K. A., MURROUGH, J. W., PEREZ, A. M., Reich, D. L., Charney, D. S., & Mathew, S. J. (2010). Safety and Efficacy of Repeated-Dose Intravenous Ketamine for Treatment-Resistant Depression. Biological Psychiatry, 67(2), 139–145. https://doi.org/10.1016/j.biopsych.2009.08.038

Abdel Azeem, A. I., Mohamed, H. S., Asida, S. M., & Ahmed, M. A. R. S. (2023). Ultra-sound guided supraclavicular brachial plexus block: The value of adjuvants: Review article. SVU-International Journal of Medical Sciences, 6(1), 312–328. https://doi.org/10.21608/svuijm.2022.159934.1399

Abreu, L. N. de, Lafer, B., Baca-Garcia, E., & Oquendo, M. A. (2009). Suicidal ideation and suicide attempts in bipolar disorder type I: an update for the clinician. Revista Brasileira de Psiquiatria, 31(3), 271–280. https://doi.org/10.1590/s1516-44462009005000003

Acevedo-Diaz, E. E., Cavanaugh, G. W., Greenstein, D., Kraus, C., Kadriu, B., Zarate, C. A., & Park, L. T. (2020). Comprehensive assessment of side effects associated with a single dose of ketamine in treatment-resistant depression. Journal of Affective Disorders, 263, 568–575. https://doi.org/10.1016/j.jad.2019.11.028

Adachi, M., Barrot, M., Autry, A. E., Theobald, D., & Monteggia, L. M. (2008). Selective Loss of Brain-Derived Neurotrophic Factor in the Dentate Gyrus Attenuates Antidepressant Efficacy. Biological Psychiatry, 63(7), 642–649. https://doi.org/10.1016/j.biopsych.2007.09.019

Adams, T. G., Bloch, M. H., & Pittenger, C. (2017). Intranasal Ketamine and Cognitive-Behavioral Therapy for Treatment-Refractory Obsessive-Compulsive Disorder. Journal of Clinical Psychopharmacology, 37(2), 269–271. https://doi.org/10.1097/jcp.0000000000000659

Addiction Support Groups - Addiction Center. (n.d.). Addiction-Center. https://www.addictioncenter.com/treatment/support-groups/

Aizawa, E., Tsuji, H., Asahara, T., Takahashi, T., Teraishi, T., Yoshida, S., Koga, N., Hattori, K., Ota, M., & Kunugi, H. (2019). Bifidobacterium and Lactobacillus Counts in the Gut Microbiota of Patients With Bipolar Disorder and Healthy Controls. Frontiers in Psychiatry, 9. https://doi.org/10.3389/fpsyt.2018.00730

Alexandrine Corriger, & Pickering, G. (2019). Ketamine and depression: a narrative review. Drug Design Development and Therapy, Volume 13, 3051–3067. https://doi.org/10.2147/dddt.s221437

American Psychiatric Association Diagnostic and Statistical Manual of Mental Disorders (DSM-IV). (2013). SpringerReference. https://doi.org/10.1007/springerreference_179660

Anand, A., Charney, D. S., Oren, D. A., Berman, R. M., Hu, X. S., Cappiello, A., & Krystal, J. H. (2000). Attenuation of the Neuropsychiatric Effects of Ketamine With Lamotrigine. Archives of

General Psychiatry, 57(3), 270. https://doi.org/10.1001/archpsyc.57.3.270

Anderson, L. (2014, May 18). Ketamine Abuse. Drugs.com; Drugs.com. https://www.drugs.com/illicit/ketamine.html

Anxiety Drugs (Anxiolytics) Side Effects, List of Names & Interactions. (n.d.). MedicineNet. https://www.medicinenet.com/anxiolytics_for_anxiety_drug_class/article.htm

Backonja, M., Arndt, G., Gombar, K. A., Check, B., & Zimmermann, M. (1994). Response of chronic neuropathic pain syndromes to ketamine: a preliminary study. Pain, 56(1), 51–57. https://doi.org/10.1016/0304-3959(94)90149-x

Baldessarini, R. J., Pompili, M., & Tondo, L. (2006). Suicide in Bipolar Disorder: Risks and Management. CNS Spectrums, 11(6), 465–471. https://doi.org/10.1017/s1092852900014681

Bandeira, I. D., Lins-Silva, D. H., Cavenaghi, V. B., Dorea-Bandeira, I., Faria-Guimarães, D., Barouh, J. L., Jesus-Nunes, A. P., Beanes, G., Souza, L. S., Leal, G. C., Sanacora, G., Miguel, E. C., Sampaio, A. S., & Quarantini, L. C. (2022). Ketamine in the Treatment of Obsessive-Compulsive Disorder: A Systematic Review. Harvard Review of Psychiatry, 30(2), 135. https://doi.org/10.1097/HRP.0000000000000330

Banov, M. D., Young, J. R., Dunn, T., & Szabo, S. T. (2020). Efficacy and safety of ketamine in the management of anxiety and anxiety spectrum disorders: a review of the literature. CNS Spectrums, 25(3), 331–342. https://doi.org/10.1017/S1092852919001238

Banwari, G., Desai, P., & Patidar, P. (2015). Ketamine-induced affective switch in a patient with treatment-resistant depression. Indian Journal of Pharmacology, 47(4), 454. https://doi.org/10.4103/0253-7613.161277

Bartoli, F., Riboldi, I., Crocamo, C., Di Brita, C., Clerici, M., & Carrà, G. (2017). Ketamine as a rapid-acting agent for suicidal ideation: A meta-analysis. Neuroscience & Biobehavioral Reviews, 77, 232–236. https://doi.org/10.1016/j.neubiorev.2017.03.010

Bashkim Kadriu, Deng, Z., Kraus, C., Henter, I. D., & Lisanby, S. H. (2020). Not So Fast. The Journal of Clinical Psychiatry, 81(4). https://doi.org/10.4088/jcp.19ac13138

Berger, W., Mendlowicz, M. V., Marques-Portella, C., Kinrys, G., Fontenelle, L. F., Marmar, C. R., & Figueira, I. (2009). Pharmacologic alternatives to antidepressants in posttraumatic stress disorder: A systematic review. Progress in Neuro-Psychopharmacology and Biological Psychiatry, 33(2), 169–180. https://doi.org/10.1016/j.pnpbp.2008.12.004

Berman, R. M., Cappiello, A., Anand, A., Oren, D. A., Heninger, G. R., Charney, D. S., & Krystal, J. H. (2000). Antidepressant effects of ketamine in depressed patients. Biological Psychiatry, 47(4), 351–354. https://doi.org/10.1016/s0006-3223(99)00230-9

Beurel, E., Song, L., & Jope, R. S. (2011). Inhibition of glycogen synthase kinase-3 is necessary for the rapid antidepressant effect of ketamine in mice. Molecular Psychiatry, 16(11), 1068–1070. https://doi.org/10.1038/mp.2011.47

Bisaga, A., & Popik, P. (2000). In search of a new pharmacological treatment for drug and alcohol addiction: N-methyl-d-aspartate (NMDA) antagonists. Drug and Alcohol Dependence, 59(1), 1–15. https://doi.org/10.1016/s0376-8716(99)00107-6

Björkholm, C., & Monteggia, L. M. (2016). BDNF – a key transducer of antidepressant effects. Neuropharmacology, 102, 72–79. https://doi.org/10.1016/j.neuropharm.2015.10.034

Bloch, M. H., Landeros-Weisenberger, A., Kelmendi, B., Coric, V., Bracken, M. B., & Leckman, J. F. (2006). A systematic review: antipsychotic augmentation with treatment refractory obsessive-compulsive disorder. Molecular Psychiatry, 11(7), 622–632. https://doi.org/10.1038/sj.mp.4001823

Bloch, M. H., McGuire, J., Landeros-Weisenberger, A., Leckman, J. F., & Pittenger, C. (2009). Meta-analysis of the dose-response relationship of SSRI in obsessive-compulsive disorder. Molecular Psychiatry, 15(8), 850–855. https://doi.org/10.1038/mp.2009.50

Bloch, M. H., Wasylink, S., Landeros-Weisenberger, A., Panza, K. E., Billingslea, E., Leckman, J. F., Krystal, J. H., Bhagwagar, Z., Sanacora, G., & Pittenger, C. (2012). Effects of Ketamine in Treatment-Refractory Obsessive-Compulsive Disorder. Biological Psychiatry, 72(11), 964–970. https://doi.org/10.1016/j.biopsych.2012.05.028

Bollini, P., Pampallona, S., Tibaldi, G., Kupelnick, B., & Munizza, C. (1999). Effectiveness of antidepressants. Meta-analysis of dose-effect relationships in randomised clinical trials. The British Journal of Psychiatry: The Journal of Mental Science, 174, 297–303. https://doi.org/10.1192/bjp.174.4.297

Brazier, Y. (2020, September 3). Suicidal ideation: Symptoms, causes, prevention, and resources. Www.medicalnewstoday.com. https://www.medicalnewstoday.com/articles/193026

Breslau, N. (1992). Migraine, suicidal ideation, and suicide attempts. Neurology, 42(2), 392–392. https://doi.org/10.1212/wnl.42.2.392

Brian Miller, M. D. (2020). Schizophrenia and AUD. Www.psychiatrictimes.com, 37. https://www.psychiatrictimes.com/view/schizophrenia-aud

Browne, C. A., Jacobson, M. L., & Lucki, I. (2020). Novel Targets to Treat Depression: Opioid-Based Therapeutics. Harvard Review of Psychiatry, 28(1), 40–59. https://doi.org/10.1097/hrp.0000000000000242

Burma, N. E., Kwok, C. H., & Trang, T. (2017). Therapies and mechanisms of opioid withdrawal. Pain Management, 7(6), 455–459. https://doi.org/10.2217/pmt-2017-0028

Byers, A. L., & Yaffe, K. (2011). Depression and risk of developing dementia. Nature Reviews Neurology, 7(6), 323–331. https://doi.org/10.1038/nrneurol.2011.60

Byers, A. L., Yaffe, K., Covinsky, K. E., Friedman, M. B., & Bruce, M. L. (2010). High Occurrence of Mood and Anxiety Disorders Among Older Adults. Archives of General Psychiatry, 67(5), 489. https://doi.org/10.1001/archgenpsychiatry.2010.35

Caddy, C., Amit, B. H., McCloud, T. L., Rendell, J. M., Furukawa, T. A., McShane, R., Hawton, K., & Cipriani, A. (2015). Ketamine and other glutamate receptor modulators for depression in adults. Cochrane Database of Systematic Reviews. https://doi.org/10.1002/14651858.cd011612.pub2

Carmin, C. N., Wiegartz, P. S., Yunus, U., & Gillock, K. L. (2002). Treatment of late-onset OCD following basal ganglia infarct. Depression and Anxiety, 15(2), 87–90. https://doi.org/10.1002/da.10024

Cate Carter, T. D., Mundo, E., Parikh, S. V., & Kennedy, J. L. (2003). Early age at onset as a risk factor for poor outcome of bipolar disorder. Journal of Psychiatric Research, 37(4), 297–303. https://doi.org/10.1016/s0022-3956(03)00052-9

Cavalli, E., Mammana, S., Nicoletti, F., Bramanti, P., & Mazzon, E. (2019). The neuropathic pain: An overview of the current treatment and future therapeutic approaches. International Journal of Immunopathology and Pharmacology, 33(33), 205873841983838. https://doi.org/10.1177/2058738419838383

Chambers, R. A., Bremner, J. D., Moghaddam, B., Southwick, S. M., Charney, D. S., & Krystal, J. H. (1999). Glutamate and post-traumatic stress disorder: toward a psychobiology of dissociation. Seminars in Clinical Neuropsychiatry, 4(4), 274–281. https://doi.org/ 10.153/SCNP00400274

Chazan, RN, S., Ekstein, MD, M. P., Marouani, MD, N., & Weinbroum, MD, A. A. (2018). Ketamine for acute and subacute pain in opioid-tolerant patients. Journal of Opioid Management, 4(3), 173. https://doi.org/10.5055/jom.2008.0023

Chen, M.-H., Li, C.-T., Lin, W.-C., Hong, C.-J., Tu, P.-C., Bai, Y.-M., Cheng, C.-M., & Su, T.-P. (2018). Rapid inflammation modulation and antidepressant efficacy of a low-dose ketamine infusion in treatment-resistant depression: A randomized, double-blind control study. Psychiatry Research, 269, 207–211. https://doi.org/10. 1016/j.psychres.2018.08.078

Chen, Y., Bai, J., Wu, D., Yu, S., Qiang, X., Bai, H., Wang, H., & Peng, Z. (2019). Association between fecal microbiota and generalized anxiety disorder: Severity and early treatment response. Journal of Affective Disorders, 259, 56–66. https://doi.org/10.1016/j.jad.2019. 08.014

Cherif, F., Zouari, H. G., Cherif, W., Hadded, M., Cheour, M., & Damak, R. (2020). Depression Prevalence in Neuropathic Pain and Its Impact on the Quality of Life. Pain Research and Management, 2020, 1–8. https://doi.org/10.1155/2020/7408508

Chiu, C.-T., Scheuing, L., Liu, G., Liao, H.-M., Linares, G. R., Lin, D., & Chuang, D.-M. (2015). The Mood Stabilizer Lithium Potentiates the Antidepressant-Like Effects and Ameliorates Oxidative

Stress Induced by Acute Ketamine in a Mouse Model of Stress. International Journal of Neuropsychopharmacology, 18(6). https://doi.org/10.1093/ijnp/pyu102

Cohen, S. P., Bhatia, A., Buvanendran, A., Schwenk, E. S., Wasan, A. D., Hurley, R. W., Viscusi, E. R., Narouze, S., Davis, F. N., Ritchie, E. C., Lubenow, T. R., & Hooten, W. M. (2018). Consensus Guidelines on the Use of Intravenous Ketamine Infusions for Chronic Pain From the American Society of Regional Anesthesia and Pain Medicine, the American Academy of Pain Medicine, and the American Society of Anesthesiologists. Regional Anesthesia and Pain Medicine, 43(5), 1. https://doi.org/10.1097/aap.0000000000000808

Connery, H. S. (2015). Medication-Assisted Treatment of Opioid Use Disorder. Harvard Review of Psychiatry, 23(2), 63–75. https://doi.org/10.1097/hrp.0000000000000075

Corinne O'Keefe Osborn. (2019, April 11). How Long Does Withdrawal From Benzodiazepines Last? Verywell Mind; Verywell Mind. https://www.verywellmind.com/benzodiazepine-withdrawal-4588452

Corriger, A., & Pickering, G. (2019). Ketamine and depression: a narrative review. Drug Design, Development and Therapy, Volume 13(13), 3051–3067. https://doi.org/10.2147/dddt.s221437

Costigan, M., Scholz, J., & Woolf, C. J. (2009). Neuropathic Pain: A Maladaptive Response of the Nervous System to Damage. Annual Review of Neuroscience, 32(1), 1–32. https://doi.org/10.1146/annurev.neuro.051508.135531

Crosstalk between the microbiota-gut-brain axis and depression. (2020). Heliyon, 6(6), e04097. https://doi.org/10.1016/j.heliyon.2020.e04097

CTG Labs - NCBI. (n.d.). Clinicaltrials.gov. Retrieved October 23, 2023, from https://clinicaltrials.gov/ct2/show/NCT00961194

Cui, H., Meng, Y., & Bulleit, R. F. (1998). Inhibition of glycogen synthase kinase 3β activity regulates proliferation of cultured cerebellar granule cells. Developmental Brain Research, 111(2), 177–188. https://doi.org/10.1016/s0165-3806(98)00136-9

D'Andrea, D., & Andrew Sewell, R. (2013). Transient Resolution of Treatment-Resistant Posttraumatic Stress Disorder Following Ketamine Infusion. Biological Psychiatry, 74(9), e13–e14. https://doi.org/10.1016/j.biopsych.2013.04.019

Das, R. K., Gale, G., Walsh, K., Hennessy, V. E., Iskandar, G., Mordecai, L. A., Brandner, B., Kindt, M., Curran, H. V., & Kamboj, S. K. (2019). Ketamine can reduce harmful drinking by pharmacologically rewriting drinking memories. Nature Communications, 10(1). https://doi.org/10.1038/s41467-019-13162-w

Demchenko, I., Tassone, V. K., Kennedy, S. H., Dunlop, K., & Bhat, V. (2022). Intrinsic Connectivity Networks of Glutamate-Mediated Antidepressant Response: A Neuroimaging Review. Frontiers in Psychiatry, 13. https://doi.org/10.3389/fpsyt.2022.864902

Dementia. (n.d.). Www.who.int. https://www.who.int/news-room/fact-sheets/detail/dementia#:~:text=Dementia%20is%20a%20syndrome%20in

Deng, X.-M., Xiao, W.-J., Luo, M.-P., Tang, G.-Z., & Xu, K.-L. (2001). The Use of Midazolam and Small-Dose Ketamine for Sedation and Analgesia During Local Anesthesia. Anesthesia & Analgesia, 93(5), 1174–1177. https://doi.org/10.1097/00000539-200111000-00023

DiazGranados, N., Ibrahim, L. A., Brutsche, N. E., Ameli, R., Henter, I. D., Luckenbaugh, D. A., Machado-Vieira, R., & Zarate, C. A.

(2010). Rapid Resolution of Suicidal Ideation After a Single Infusion of anN-Methyl-D-Aspartate Antagonist in Patients With Treatment-Resistant Major Depressive Disorder. The Journal of Clinical Psychiatry, 71(12), 1605–1611. https://doi.org/10.4088/jcp.09m05327blu

Diazgranados, N., Ibrahim, L., Brutsche, N. E., Newberg, A., Kronstein, P., Khalife, S., Kammerer, W. A., Quezado, Z., Luckenbaugh, D. A., Salvadore, G., Machado-Vieira, R., Manji, H. K., & Zarate, C. A. (2010). A Randomized Add-on Trial of an N-methyl-D-aspartate Antagonist in Treatment-Resistant Bipolar Depression. Archives of General Psychiatry, 67(8), 793. https://doi.org/10.1001/archgenpsychiatry.2010.90

Domènech, L., Willis, J., Alemany-Navarro, M., Morell, M., Real, E., Escaramís, G., Bertolín, S., Sánchez Chinchilla, D., Balcells, S., Segalàs, C., Estivill, X., Menchón, J. M., Gabaldón, T., Alonso, P., & Rabionet, R. (2022). Changes in the stool and oropharyngeal microbiome in obsessive-compulsive disorder. Scientific Reports, 12(1), 1448. https://doi.org/10.1038/s41598-022-05480-9

Domino, E. F. (2010). Taming the Ketamine Tiger. Anesthesiology, 113(3), 1. https://doi.org/10.1097/aln.0b013e3181ed09a2

Drugs & Medications. (2019). Webmd.com. https://www.webmd.com/drugs/2/drug-920-6006/klonopin-oral/clonazepam-oral/details

Duman, R. S., Sanacora, G., & Krystal, J. H. (2019). Altered Connectivity in Depression: GABA and Glutamate Neurotransmitter Deficits and Reversal by Novel Treatments. Neuron, 102(1), 75–90. https://doi.org/10.1016/j.neuron.2019.03.013

Eaton, W. W., Shao, H., Nestadt, G., Lee, B. H., Bienvenu, O. J., & Zandi, P. (2008). Population-Based Study of First Onset and Chronicity in Major Depressive Disorder. Archives of General Psychiatry, 65(5), 513. https://doi.org/10.1001/archpsyc.65.5.513

Edinoff, A. N., Hegefeld, T. L., Petersen, M., Patterson, J. C., Yossi, C., Slizewski, J., Osumi, A., Cornett, E. M., Kaye, A., Kaye, J. S., Javalkar, V., Viswanath, O., Urits, I., & Kaye, A. D. (2022). Transcranial Magnetic Stimulation for Post-traumatic Stress Disorder. Frontiers in Psychiatry, 13. https://doi.org/10.3389/fpsyt.2022. 701348

Feder, A., Costi, S., Rutter, S. B., Collins, A. B., Govindarajulu, U., Jha, M. K., Horn, S. R., Kautz, M., Corniquel, M., Collins, K. A., Bevilacqua, L., Glasgow, A. M., Brallier, J., Pietrzak, R. H., Murrough, J. W., & Charney, D. S. (2021). A Randomized Controlled Trial of Repeated Ketamine Administration for Chronic Posttraumatic Stress Disorder. American Journal of Psychiatry, 178(2), 193–202. https://doi.org/10.1176/appi.ajp.2020. 20050596

Feder, A., Parides, M. K., Murrough, J. W., Perez, A. M., Morgan, J. E., Saxena, S., Kirkwood, K., aan het Rot, M., Lapidus, K. A. B., Wan, L.-B., Iosifescu, D., & Charney, D. S. (2014). Efficacy of Intravenous Ketamine for Treatment of Chronic Posttraumatic Stress Disorder. JAMA Psychiatry, 71(6), 681. https://doi.org/10.1001/ jamapsychiatry.2014.62

Feifel, D., Malcolm, B., Boggie, D., & Lee, K. (2017). Low-dose ketamine for treatment resistant depression in an academic clinical practice setting. Journal of Affective Disorders, 221, 283–288. https://doi.org/10.1016/j.jad.2017.06.043

Filho, C. B., Jesse, C. R., Donato, F., Giacomeli, R., Del Fabbro, L., da Silva Antunes, M., de Gomes, M. G., Goes, A. T. R., Boeira, S. P., Prigol, M., & Souza, L. C. (2015). Chronic unpredictable mild stress decreases BDNF and NGF levels and Na(+),K(+)-ATPase activity in the hippocampus and prefrontal cortex of mice: antidepressant effect of chrysin. Neuroscience, 289, 367–380. https://doi.org/10. 1016/j.neuroscience.2014.12.048

Foa, E. B., Liebowitz, M. R., Kozak, M. J., Davies, S., Campeas, R., Franklin, M. E., Huppert, J. D., Kjernisted, K., Rowan, V., Schmidt, A. B., Simpson, H. B., & Tu, X. (2005). Randomized, Placebo-Controlled Trial of Exposure and Ritual Prevention, Clomipramine, and Their Combination in the Treatment of Obsessive-Compulsive Disorder. American Journal of Psychiatry, 162(1), 151–161. https://doi.org/10.1176/appi.ajp.162.1.151

Frick, L., & Pittenger, C. (2016). Microglial Dysregulation in OCD, Tourette Syndrome, and PANDAS. Journal of Immunology Research, 2016, 1–8. https://doi.org/10.1155/2016/8606057

Fukumoto, K., Toki, H., Iijima, M., Hashihayata, T., Yamaguchi, J., Hashimoto, K., & Chaki, S. (2017). Antidepressant Potential of (R)-Ketamine in Rodent Models: Comparison with (S)-Ketamine . Journal of Pharmacology and Experimental Therapeutics, 361(1), 9–16. https://doi.org/10.1124/jpet.116.239228

Gagne, C., Piot, A., & Brake, W. G. (2022). Depression, Estrogens, and Neuroinflammation: A Preclinical Review of Ketamine Treatment for Mood Disorders in Women. Frontiers in Psychiatry, 12. https://doi.org/10.3389/fpsyt.2021.797577

Gamma-Aminobutyric Acid (Gaba): Uses, Side Effects, Interactions, Dosage, and Warning. (n.d.). Www.webmd.com. https://www.webmd.com/vitamins/ai/ingredientmono-464/gamma-aminobutyric-acid-gaba

Gaynes, B. N., Lux, L., Gartlehner, G., Asher, G., Forman-Hoffman, V., Green, J., Boland, E., Weber, R. P., Randolph, C., Bann, C., Coker-Schwimmer, E., Viswanathan, M., & Lohr, K. N. (2019). Defining treatment-resistant depression. Depression and Anxiety, 37(2). https://doi.org/10.1002/da.22968

Gerentes, M., Pelissolo, A., Rajagopal, K., Tamouza, R., & Hamdani, N. (2019). Obsessive-Compulsive Disorder: Autoimmunity and Neuroinflammation. Current Psychiatry Reports, 21(8). https://doi.org/10.1007/s11920-019-1062-8

Getachew, B., Aubee, J. I., Schottenfeld, R. S., Csoka, A. B., Thompson, K. M., & Tizabi, Y. (2018). Ketamine interactions with gut-microbiota in rats: relevance to its antidepressant and anti-inflammatory properties. BMC Microbiology, 18(1). https://doi.org/10.1186/s12866-018-1373-7

Grande, I., Fries, G. R., Kunz, M., & Kapczinski, F. (2010). The Role of BDNF as a Mediator of Neuroplasticity in Bipolar Disorder. Psychiatry Investigation, 7(4), 243. https://doi.org/10.4306/pi.2010.7.4.243

Grunebaum, M. F., Ellis, S. P., Keilp, J. G., Moitra, V. K., Cooper, T. B., Marver, J. E., Burke, A. K., Milak, M. S., Sublette, M. E., Oquendo, M. A., & Mann, J. J. (2017). Ketamine versus midazolam in bipolar depression with suicidal thoughts: A pilot midazolam-controlled randomized clinical trial. Bipolar Disorders, 19(3), 176–183. https://doi.org/10.1111/bdi.12487

Grunebaum, M. F., Galfalvy, H. C., Choo, T.-H., Keilp, J. G., Moitra, V. K., Parris, M. S., Marver, J. E., Burke, A. K., Milak, M. S., Sublette, M. E., Oquendo, M. A., & Mann, J. J. (2018). Ketamine for Rapid Reduction of Suicidal Thoughts in Major Depression: A Midazolam-Controlled Randomized Clinical Trial. American Journal of Psychiatry, 175(4), 327–335. https://doi.org/10.1176/appi.ajp.2017.17060647

Guillemin, G. J., Smith, D. G., Smythe, G. A., Armati, P. J., & Brew, B. J. (2003). Expression of the kynurenine pathway enzymes in human microglia and macrophages. Advances in Experimental Medicine and Biology, 527, 105–112. https://doi.org/10.1007/978-1-4615-0135-0_12

H. Bloch, M., & Pittenger, C. (2010). The Genetics of Obsessive-Compulsive Disorder. Current Psychiatry Reviews, 6(2), 91–103. https://doi.org/10.2174/157340010791196439

Hashimoto, K. (2016). Ketamine's antidepressant action: beyond NMDA receptor inhibition. Expert Opinion on Therapeutic Targets, 20(11), 1389–1392. https://doi.org/10.1080/14728222.2016.1238899

Hashimoto, K. (2019). Rapid-acting antidepressant ketamine, its metabolites and other candidates: A historical overview and future perspective. Psychiatry and Clinical Neurosciences, 73(10), 613–627. https://doi.org/10.1111/pcn.12902

Hasselmann, H. (2014). Ketamine as Antidepressant? Current State and Future Perspectives. Current Neuropharmacology, 12(1), 57–70. https://doi.org/10.2174/1570159x113119990043

Hedegaard, H., Miniño, A., & Warner, M. (2020). Drug Overdose Deaths in the United States, 1999-2018 Key findings Data from the National Vital Statistics System, Mortality. https://www.cdc.gov/nchs/data/databriefs/db356-h.pdf

Hedegaard, M., Hansen, K. B., Andersen, K. T., Bräuner-Osborne, H., & Traynelis, S. F. (2012). Molecular pharmacology of human NMDA receptors. Neurochemistry International, 61(4), 601–609. https://doi.org/10.1016/j.neuint.2011.11.016

Hidalgo, R. B., & Davidson, J. R. T. (2000). Selective serotonin reuptake inhibitors in post-traumatic stress disorder. Journal of Psychopharmacology, 14(1), 70–76. https://doi.org/10.1177/026988110001400110

Hodgman-Korth, M. (2022, January 7). The Side Effects of Ketamine - Treatment Options. American Addiction Centers. https://

americanaddictioncenters.org/ketamine-abuse/ketamine-side-effects

How Do NMDA Antagonists Work? Uses, Side Effects, Drug Names. (n.d.). RxList. https://www.rxlist.com/nmda_antagonists/drug-class.htm

https://www.facebook.com/Drugscom. (2019). Lamictal. Drugs.com; Drugs.com. https://www.drugs.com/lamictal.html

https://www.facebook.com/NIHAging. (2014, May 22). Number of Alzheimer's deaths found to be underreported. National Institute on Aging. https://www.nia.nih.gov/news/number-alzheimers-deaths-found-be-underreported

Huang, R., Wang, K., & Hu, J. (2016). Effect of Probiotics on Depression: A Systematic Review and Meta-Analysis of Randomized Controlled Trials. Nutrients, 8(8), 483. https://doi.org/10.3390/nu8080483

Institute of Medicine (US) Forum on Neuroscience and Nervous System Disorders. (2011). Overview of the Glutamatergic System. Nih.gov; National Academies Press (US). https://www.ncbi.nlm.nih.gov/books/NBK62187/

IV Ketamine Infusions Dramatically Improve the Quality of Life for Severe Migraine Patient. (n.d.). BioSpace. Retrieved October 23, 2023, from https://www.biospace.com/article/releases/iv-ketamine-infusions-dramatically-improve-the-quality-of-life-for-severe-migraine-patient/

Jacobs, S. (2020, August 10). IV Ketamine for Adults With MDD or Bipolar Disorder: Safety and Tolerability. Psychiatry Advisor. https://www.psychiatryadvisor.com/home/depression-advisor/iv-ketamine-for-adults-with-mdd-or-bipolar-disorder-safety-and-tolerability/

Jamison, K. R. (2000). Suicide and bipolar disorder. The Journal of Clinical Psychiatry, 61 Suppl 9, 47–51. https://pubmed.ncbi.nlm.nih.gov/10826661/

Jeon, W. J., Dean, B., Scarr, E., & Gibbons, A. (2015). The Role of Muscarinic Receptors in the Pathophysiology of Mood Disorders: A Potential Novel Treatment? Current Neuropharmacology, 13(6), 739–749. https://doi.org/10.2174/1570159X13666150612230045

Jesulola, E., Micalos, P., & Baguley, I. J. (2018). Understanding the pathophysiology of depression: From monoamines to the neurogenesis hypothesis model - are we there yet? Behavioural Brain Research, 341, 79–90. https://doi.org/10.1016/j.bbr.2017.12.025

Jones, J. L., Mateus, C. F., Malcolm, R. J., Brady, K. T., & Back, S. E. (2018). Efficacy of Ketamine in the Treatment of Substance Use Disorders: A Systematic Review. Frontiers in Psychiatry, 9. https://doi.org/10.3389/fpsyt.2018.00277

Jovaisa, T., Laurinenas, G., Vosylius, S., Sipylaite, J., Badaras, R., & Ivaskevicius, J. (2006). Effects of ketamine on precipitated opiate withdrawal. Medicina (Kaunas, Lithuania), 42(8), 625–634. https://pubmed.ncbi.nlm.nih.gov/16963828/

Kadriu, B., Farmer, C. A., Yuan, P., Park, L. T., Deng, Z.-D., Moaddel, R., Henter, I. D., Shovestul, B., Ballard, E. D., Kraus, C., Gold, P. W., Machado-Vieira, R., & Zarate, C. A. (2019). The kynurenine pathway and bipolar disorder: intersection of the monoaminergic and glutamatergic systems and immune response. Molecular Psychiatry. https://doi.org/10.1038/s41380-019-0589-8

Kadriu, B., Musazzi, L., Henter, I. D., Graves, M., Popoli, M., & Zarate, C. A. (2019). Glutamatergic Neurotransmission: Pathway to Developing Novel Rapid-Acting Antidepressant Treatments. International Journal of Neuropsychopharmacology, 22(2), 119–135. https://doi.org/10.1093/ijnp/pyy094

Katalinic, N., Lai, R., Somogyi, A., Mitchell, P. B., Glue, P., & Loo, C. K. (2013). Ketamine as a new treatment for depression: A review of its efficacy and adverse effects. Australian & New Zealand Journal of Psychiatry, 47(8), 710–727. https://doi.org/10.1177/0004867413486842

Kator, S., Correll, D. J., Ou, J. Y., Levinson, R., Noronha, G. N., & Adams, C. D. (2016). Assessment of low-dose i.v. ketamine infusions for adjunctive analgesia. American Journal of Health-System Pharmacy, 73(5_Supplement_1), S22–S29. https://doi.org/10.2146/ajhp150367

Kaufman, J., & Charney, D. (2000). Comorbidity of mood and anxiety disorders. Depression and Anxiety, 12 Suppl 1, 69–76. https://doi.org/10.1002/1520-6394(2000)12:1+3.0.CO;2-K

Ketalar (ketamine) dosing, indications, interactions, adverse effects, and more. (n.d.). Reference.medscape.com. https://reference.medscape.com/drug/ketalar-ketamine-343099#3

Ketamine and Xanax Interactions Checker. (n.d.). Drugs.com. Retrieved October 23, 2023, from https://www.drugs.com/drug-interactions/ketamine-with-xanax-1411-0-133-54.html?professional=1

Ketamine for Depression and Mood Disorders. (n.d.). Townsend Letter. https://www.townsendletter.com/article/438-ketamine-for-depression-and-mood-disorders/

Ketamine May Help People with Alcohol Use Disorder. (2022, January 11). Healthline. https://www.healthline.com/health-news/ketamine-and-psychological-therapy-may-help-people-with-severe-alcohol-use-disorder

Ketamine Migraine Treatment. (2017, November 2). Healthline. https://www.healthline.com/health-news/can-ketamine-reduce-the-pain-of-migraines

Ketamine Research in Russia. (n.d.). Maps.org. Retrieved October 23, 2023, from https://maps.org/research-archive/ketamine/ketrussi a.html

Ketamine: A Transformational Catalyst. (2016, December 2). Multidisciplinary Association for Psychedelic Studies - MAPS. https://maps.org/news/bulletin/articles/410-bulletin-winter-2016/ 6470-ketamine-a-transformational-catalyst

Kiraly, D. D., Horn, S. R., Van Dam, N. T., Costi, S., Schwartz, J., Kim-Schulze, S., Patel, M., Hodes, G. E., Russo, S. J., Merad, M., Iosifescu, D. V., Charney, D. S., & Murrough, J. W. (2017). Altered peripheral immune profiles in treatment-resistant depression: response to ketamine and prediction of treatment outcome. Translational Psychiatry, 7(3), e1065. https://doi.org/10.1038/tp.2017.31

Kishimoto, T., Chawla, J. M., Hagi, K., Zarate, C. A., Kane, J. M., Bauer, M., & Correll, C. U. (2016). Single-dose infusion ketamine and non-ketamine N-methyl-d-aspartate receptor antagonists for unipolar and bipolar depression: a meta-analysis of efficacy, safety and time trajectories. Psychological Medicine, 46(7), 1459–1472. https://doi.org/10.1017/s0033291716000064

Kitching, D. (2015). Depression in dementia. Australian Prescriber, 38(6), 209–211. https://doi.org/10.18773/austprescr.2015.071

Kozlovskii, V. L., Popov, M. Yu., Kosterin, D. N., & Lepik, O. V. (2021). Heterogeneity of the mechanisms of action of antidepressants. V.M. BEKHTEREV REVIEW of PSYCHIATRY and MEDICAL PSYCHOLOGY, 1, 11–17. https://doi.org/10.31363/2313-7053-2021-1-11-17

Kraus, C., Wasserman, D., Henter, I. D., Acevedo-Diaz, E., Kadriu, B., & Zarate, C. A. (2019). The influence of ketamine on drug discovery in depression. Drug Discovery Today, 24(10), 2033–2043. https://doi.org/10.1016/j.drudis.2019.07.007

Krupitsky, E. M., & Grinenko, A. Y. (1997). Ketamine Psychedelic Therapy (KPT): A Review of the Results of Ten Years of Research. Journal of Psychoactive Drugs, 29(2), 165–183. https://doi.org/10.1080/02791072.1997.10400185

Krupitsky, E., Burakov, A., Romanova, T., Dunaevsky, I., Strassman, R., & Grinenko, A. (2002). Ketamine psychotherapy for heroin addiction: immediate effects and two-year follow-up. Journal of Substance Abuse Treatment, 23(4), 273–283. https://doi.org/10.1016/s0740-5472(02)00275-1

Kurdi, M. S., Theerth, K. A., & Deva, R. S. (2014). Ketamine: Current applications in anesthesia, pain, and critical care. Anesthesia: Essays and Researches, 8(3), 283. https://doi.org/10.4103/0259-1162.143110

Laje, G., Paddock, S., Manji, H., Rush, A. J., Wilson, A. F., Charney, D., & McMahon, F. J. (2007). Genetic Markers of Suicidal Ideation Emerging During Citalopram Treatment of Major Depression. American Journal of Psychiatry, 164(10), 1530–1538. https://doi.org/10.1176/appi.ajp.2007.06122018

Lalanne, L., Nicot, C., Lang, J.-P., Bertschy, G., & Salvat, E. (2016). Experience of the use of Ketamine to manage opioid withdrawal in an addicted woman: a case report. BMC Psychiatry, 16(1), 395. https://doi.org/10.1186/s12888-016-1112-2

Lane, H.-Y., Lu, Y.-Y., & Lin, C.-H. (2016). Mania following ketamine abuse. Neuropsychiatric Disease and Treatment, 237. https://doi.org/10.2147/ndt.s97696

Lara, D. R., Bisol, L. W., & Munari, L. R. (2013). Antidepressant, mood stabilizing and procognitive effects of very low dose sublingual ketamine in refractory unipolar and bipolar depression. The International Journal of Neuropsychopharmacology, 16(09), 2111–2117. https://doi.org/10.1017/s1461145713000485

Larkin, G. L., & Beautrais, A. L. (2011). A preliminary naturalistic study of low-dose ketamine for depression and suicide ideation in the emergency department. International Journal of Neuropsychopharmacology, 14(8), 1127–1131. https://doi.org/10.1017/s1461145711000629

Lauritsen, C., Mazuera, S., Lipton, R. B., & Ashina, S. (2016). Intravenous ketamine for subacute treatment of refractory chronic migraine: a case series. The Journal of Headache and Pain, 17(1). https://doi.org/10.1186/s10194-016-0700-3

Leckman, J. F., Goodman, W. K., North, W. G., Chappell, P. B., Price, L. H., Pauls, D. L., Anderson, G. M., Riddle, M. A., McSwiggan-Hardin, M., McDougle, C. J., Barr, L. C., & Cohen, D. J. (1994). Elevated Cerebrospinal Fluid Levels of Oxytocin in Obsessive-compulsive Disorder: Comparison With Tourette's Syndrome and Healthy Controls. Archives of General Psychiatry, 51(10), 782–792. https://doi.org/10.1001/archpsyc.1994.03950100030003

Ledesma, P. (2020, January 2). How Much Does a Clinical Trial Cost? Sofpromed. https://www.sofpromed.com/how-much-does-a-clinical-trial-cost/

Lester, H. A., Lavis, L. D., & Dougherty, D. A. (2015). Ketamine Inside Neurons? The American Journal of Psychiatry, 172(11), 1064–1066. https://doi.org/10.1176/appi.ajp.2015.14121537

Li, L., & Vlisides, P. E. (2016). Ketamine: 50 Years of Modulating the Mind. Frontiers in Human Neuroscience, 10(612). https://doi.org/10.3389/fnhum.2016.00612

Liriano, F., Hatten, C., & Schwartz, T. L. (2019). Ketamine as treatment for post-traumatic stress disorder: a review. Drugs in Context, 8, 1–7. https://doi.org/10.7573/dic.212305

Long Term Effects of Chronic Migraine. (n.d.). TheraSpecs. Retrieved February 26, 2023, from https://www.theraspecs.com/blog/long-term-effects-chronic-migraine/

LSW, B. S. Y., MA. (2018, February 19). Ketamine: A Promising Agent for Managing Treatment-Resistant Depression. Psychiatry Advisor. https://www.psychiatryadvisor.com/home/depression-advisor/ketamine-a-promising-agent-for-managing-treatment-resistant-depression/

Ludwig, B., & Dwivedi, Y. (2016). Dissecting bipolar disorder complexity through epigenomic approach. Molecular Psychiatry, 21(11), 1490–1498. https://doi.org/10.1038/mp.2016.123

Luscher, B., Shen, Q., & Sahir, N. (2010). The GABAergic deficit hypothesis of major depressive disorder. Molecular Psychiatry, 16(4), 383–406. https://doi.org/10.1038/mp.2010.120

Macedo, D., Filho, A. J. M. C., Soares de Sousa, C. N., Quevedo, J., Barichello, T., Júnior, H. V. N., & Freitas de Lucena, D. (2017). Antidepressants, antimicrobials or both? Gut microbiota dysbiosis in depression and possible implications of the antimicrobial effects of antidepressant drugs for antidepressant effectiveness. Journal of Affective Disorders, 208, 22–32. https://doi.org/10.1016/j.jad.2016.09.012

Machado-Vieira, R., Gold, P. W., Luckenbaugh, D. A., Ballard, E. D., Richards, E. M., Henter, I. D., De Sousa, R. T., Niciu, M. J., Yuan, P., & Zarate, C. A. (2016). The role of adipokines in the rapid antidepressant effects of ketamine. Molecular Psychiatry, 22(1), 127–133. https://doi.org/10.1038/mp.2016.36

Machado-Vieira, R., Ibrahim, L., & Zarate Jr., C. A. (2010). Histone Deacetylases and Mood Disorders: Epigenetic Programming in Gene-Environment Interactions. CNS Neuroscience & Therapeutics, 17(6), 699–704. https://doi.org/10.1111/j.1755-5949.2010.00203.x

Maher, D. P., Chen, L., & Mao, J. (2017). Intravenous Ketamine Infusions for Neuropathic Pain Management. Anesthesia & Analgesia, 124(2), 661–674. https://doi.org/10.1213/ane.0000000000001787

Makin, S. (2019, April 12). Behind the Buzz: How Ketamine Changes the Depressed Patient's Brain. Scientific American. https://www.scientificamerican.com/article/behind-the-buzz-how-ketamine-changes-the-depressed-patients-brain/

Malhotra, M.D., A. (1997). Ketamine-Induced Exacerbation of Psychotic Symptoms and Cognitive Impairment in Neuroleptic-Free Schizophrenics. Neuropsychopharmacology, 17(3), 141–150. https://doi.org/10.1016/s0893-133x(97)00036-5

Marijn Lijffijt, Green, C. E., Balderston, N. L., Iqbal, T., Atkinson, M., Vo-Le, B., Bylinda Vo-Le, O'Brien, B., Grillon, C., Swann, A. C., & Mathew, S. J. (2019). A Proof-of-Mechanism Study to Test Effects of the NMDA Receptor Antagonist Lanicemine on Behavioral Sensitization in Individuals With Symptoms of PTSD. Frontiers in Psychiatry, 10. https://doi.org/10.3389/fpsyt.2019.00846

Martinotti, G., Chiappini, S., Pettorruso, M., Mosca, A., Miuli, A., Di Carlo, F., D'Andrea, G., Collevecchio, R., Di Muzio, I., Sensi, S. L., & Di Giannantonio, M. (2021). Therapeutic Potentials of Ketamine and Esketamine in Obsessive–Compulsive Disorder (OCD), Substance Use Disorders (SUD) and Eating Disorders (ED): A Review of the Current Literature. Brain Sciences, 11(7), 856. https://doi.org/10.3390/brainsci11070856

Matveychuk, D., Thomas, R. K., Swainson, J., Khullar, A., MacKay, M.-A., Baker, G. B., & Dursun, S. M. (2020). Ketamine as an antidepressant: overview of its mechanisms of action and potential predictive biomarkers. Therapeutic Advances in Psychopharmacology, 10, 204512532091665. https://doi.org/10.1177/2045125320916657

McGowan, J. C., LaGamma, C. T., Lim, S. C., Tsitsiklis, M., Neria, Y., Brachman, R. A., & Denny, C. A. (2017). Prophylactic Ketamine Attenuates Learned Fear. Neuropsychopharmacology, 42(8), 1577–1589. https://doi.org/10.1038/npp.2017.19

McIntyre, R. S., Rodrigues, N. B., Lee, Y., Lipsitz, O., Subramaniapillai, M., Gill, H., Nasri, F., Majeed, A., Lui, L. M. W., Senyk, O., Phan, L., Carvalho, I. P., Siegel, A., Mansur, R. B., Brietzke, E., Kratiuk, K., Arekapudi, A. K., Abrishami, A., Chau, E. H., & Szpejda, W. (2020). The effectiveness of repeated intravenous ketamine on depressive symptoms, suicidal ideation and functional disability in adults with major depressive disorder and bipolar disorder: Results from the Canadian Rapid Treatment Center of Excellence. Journal of Affective Disorders, 274, 903–910. https://doi.org/10.1016/j.jad.2020.05.088

McNicholas, L. F. (2010). Poster Abstracts from the AAAP 20th Annual Meeting and Symposium. American Journal on Addictions, no-no. https://doi.org/10.1111/j.1521-0391.2010.00059.x

migraineresearchfoundation.org - migraineresearchfoundation Resources and Information. (n.d.). Migraineresearchfoundation.org. Retrieved October 23, 2023, from https://migraineresearch foundation.org/about-migraine/migraine-facts/#:~:text=Nearly%201%20in%204%20U.S

Mihaljevic, S., Pavlovic, M., Reine, K., & Cacic, M. (2020). THERAPEUTIC MECHANISMS OF KETAMINE. Psychiatria Danubina, 32(3-4), 325–333. https://doi.org/10.24869/psyd.2020.325

Mion, G., & Villevieille, T. (2013). Ketamine Pharmacology: An Update (Pharmacodynamics and Molecular Aspects, Recent Findings). CNS Neuroscience & Therapeutics, 19(6), 370–380. https://doi.org/10.1111/cns.12099

Moda-Sava, R. N., Murdock, M. H., Parekh, P. K., Fetcho, R. N., Huang, B. S., Huynh, T. N., J. Witztum, Shaver, D. C., Rosenthal, D. L., Alway, E. J., K. Lopez, Y. Meng, L. Nellissen, L. Grosenick, Milner, T. A., K. Deisseroth, H. Bito, H. Kasai, & C. Liston. (2019). Sustained rescue of prefrontal circuit dysfunction by antidepressant-induced spine formation. Science, 364(6436). https://doi.org/10.1126/science.aat8078

Modabbernia, A., Taslimi, S., Brietzke, E., & Ashrafi, M. (2013). Cytokine Alterations in Bipolar Disorder: A Meta-Analysis of 30 Studies. Biological Psychiatry, 74(1), 15–25. https://doi.org/10.1016/j.biopsych.2013.01.007

Munkholm, K., Vinberg, M., Berk, M., & Kessing, L. V. (2012). State-related alterations of gene expression in bipolar disorder: a systematic review. Bipolar Disorders, 14(7), 684–696. https://doi.org/10.1111/bdi.12005

Murrough, J. W., Iosifescu, D. V., Chang, L. C., Al Jurdi, R. K., Green, C. E., Perez, A. M., Iqbal, S., Pillemer, S., Foulkes, A., Shah, A., Charney, D. S., & Mathew, S. J. (2013). Antidepressant Efficacy of Ketamine in Treatment-Resistant Major Depression: A Two-Site Randomized Controlled Trial. American Journal of Psychiatry, 170(10), 1134–1142. https://doi.org/10.1176/appi.ajp.2013.13030392

Murrough, J. W., Soleimani, L., DeWilde, K. E., Collins, K. A., Lapidus, K. A., Iacoviello, B. M., Lener, M., Kautz, M., Kim, J., Stern, J. B., Price, R. B., Perez, A. M., Brallier, J. W., Rodriguez, G. J., Goodman, W. K., Iosifescu, D. V., & Charney, D. S. (2015). Ketamine for rapid reduction of suicidal ideation: a randomized controlled trial. Psychological Medicine, 45(16), 3571–3580. https://doi.org/10.1017/s0033291715001506

Nall, R. (2015, August 24). Everything You Want to Know About Migraine. Healthline; Healthline Media. https://www.healthline.com/health/migraine

National Institute of Mental Health. (2003). Obsessive-Compulsive Disorder (OCD). Www.nimh.nih.gov. https://www.nimh.nih.gov/health/statistics/obsessive-compulsive-disorder-ocd

National Institute of Mental Health. (2017, November). NIMH» Bipolar Disorder. Nih.gov. https://www.nimh.nih.gov/health/statistics/bipolar-disorder.shtml

National Institute of Mental Health. (2022). Bipolar Disorder. Www.nimh.nih.gov. https://www.nimh.nih.gov/health/statistics/bipolar-disorder

National Institute of Neurological Disorders and Stroke. (2018, August 11). Peripheral Neuropathy Fact Sheet | National Institute of Neurological Disorders and Stroke. Nih.gov. https://www.ninds.nih.gov/Disorders/Patient-Caregiver-Education/Fact-Sheets/Peripheral-Neuropathy-Fact-Sheet

National Institute on Aging. (2023, April 5). Alzheimer's Disease Fact Sheet. National Institute on Aging. https://www.nia.nih.gov/health/alzheimers-disease-fact-sheet

Newport, D. J., Carpenter, L. L., McDonald, W. M., Potash, J. B., Tohen, M., & Nemeroff, C. B. (2015). Ketamine and Other NMDA Antagonists: Early Clinical Trials and Possible Mechanisms in Depression. American Journal of Psychiatry, 172(10), 950–966. https://doi.org/10.1176/appi.ajp.2015.15040465

Niciu, M. J., Luckenbaugh, D. A., Ionescu, D. F., Guevara, S., Machado-Vieira, R., Richards, E. M., Brutsche, N. E., Nolan, N. M., & Zarate, C. A. (2014). Clinical Predictors of Ketamine Response in Treatment-Resistant Major Depression. The Journal of Clinical Psychiatry, 75(05), e417–e423. https://doi.org/10.4088/jcp.13m08698

Niciu, M. J., Luckenbaugh, D. A., Ionescu, D. F., Richards, E. M., Vande Voort, J. L., Ballard, E. D., Brutsche, N. E., Furey, M. L., & Zarate, C. A. (2014). Ketamine's Antidepressant Efficacy is Extended for at Least Four Weeks in Subjects with a Family History of an Alcohol Use Disorder. International Journal of Neuropsychopharmacology, 18(1). https://doi.org/10.1093/ijnp/pyu039

Niesters, M., Martini, C., & Dahan, A. (2014). Ketamine for chronic pain: risks and benefits. British Journal of Clinical Pharmacology, 77(2), 357–367. https://doi.org/10.1111/bcp.12094

NIMH» Suicide in America: Frequently Asked Questions. (2019, March 28). Nih.gov. https://www.nimh.nih.gov/health/publications/suicide-faq/index.shtml

NPR Choice page. (2019). Npr.org. https://www.npr.org/sections/health-shots/2019/03/05/700509903/fda-clears-esketamine-nasal-spray-for-hard-to-treat-depression

O'Brien, S. L., Pangarkar, S., & Prager, J. (2014). The Use of Ketamine in Neuropathic Pain. Current Physical Medicine and Rehabilitation Reports, 2(2), 128–145. https://doi.org/10.1007/s40141-014-0045-2

Office of the Commissioner. (2019, March 5). FDA approves new nasal spray medication for treatment-resistant depression; available only at a certified doctor's office or clinic. U.S. Food and Drug Administration. https://www.fda.gov/news-events/press-announcements/fda-approves-new-nasal-spray-medication-treatment-resistant-depression-available-only-certified

Perez-Caballero, L., Perez, V., & Berrocoso, E. (2020). What ketamine can teach us about the opioid system in depression? Expert Opinion on Drug Discovery, 1–4. https://doi.org/10.1080/17460441.2020.1781812

Philip, N. S., Carpenter, L. L., Tyrka, A. R., & Price, L. H. (2010). Nicotinic acetylcholine receptors and depression: a review of the preclinical and clinical literature. Psychopharmacology, 212(1), 1–12. https://doi.org/10.1007/s00213-010-1932-6

Phillips, J. L., Norris, S., Talbot, J., Hatchard, T., Ortiz, A., Birmingham, M., Owoeye, O., Batten, L. A., & Blier, P. (2019). Single and repeated ketamine infusions for reduction of suicidal ideation in treatment-resistant depression. Neuropsychopharmacology. https://doi.org/10.1038/s41386-019-0570-x

Pigott, T. A., L'Heureux, F., Dubbert, B., Bernstein, S., & Murphy, D. L. (1994). Obsessive compulsive disorder: comorbid conditions. The Journal of Clinical Psychiatry, 55 Suppl, 15–27; discussion 28-32. https://pubmed.ncbi.nlm.nih.gov/7961529/

Pittenger, C., Bloch, M. H., & Williams, K. (2011). Glutamate abnormalities in obsessive compulsive disorder: Neurobiology, pathophysiology, and treatment. Pharmacology & Therapeutics, 132(3), 314–332. https://doi.org/10.1016/j.pharmthera.2011.09.006

Polomano, R. C., Buckenmaier, C. C., Kwon, K. H., Hanlon, A. L., Rupprecht, C., Goldberg, C., & Gallagher, R. M. (2013). Effects of low-dose IV ketamine on peripheral and central pain from major limb injuries sustained in combat. Pain Medicine (Malden, Mass.), 14(7), 1088–1100. https://doi.org/10.1111/pme.12094

Post-Traumatic Stress Disorder: The Management of PTSD in Adults and Children in Primary and Secondary Care. (n.d.). PubMed. https://pubmed.ncbi.nlm.nih.gov/21834189/

Price, R. B., Nock, M. K., Charney, D. S., & Mathew, S. J. (2009). Effects of Intravenous Ketamine on Explicit and Implicit Measures of Suicidality in Treatment-Resistant Depression. Biological Psychiatry, 66(5), 522–526. https://doi.org/10.1016/j. biopsych.2009.04.029

Quinlan, J. (2012). The Use of a Subanesthetic Infusion of Intravenous Ketamine to Allow Withdrawal of Medically Prescribed Opioids in People with Chronic Pain, Opioid Tolerance and Hyperalgesia: Outcome at 6 Months: Table 1. Pain Medicine, 13(11), 1524–1525. https://doi.org/10.1111/j.1526-4637.2012. 01486.x

Ramic, E., Prasko, S., Gavran, L., & Spahic, E. (2020). Assessment of the Antidepressant Side Effects Occurrence in Patients Treated in Primary Care. Materia Socio Medica, 32(2), 131. https://doi.org/ 10.5455/msm.2020.32.131-134

Rao, J. S., Harry, G. J., Rapoport, S. I., & Kim, H. W. (2009). Increased excitotoxicity and neuroinflammatory markers in post-mortem frontal cortex from bipolar disorder patients. Molecular Psychiatry, 15(4), 384–392. https://doi.org/10.1038/mp.2009.47

Ren, L., Deng, J., Min, S., Peng, L., & Chen, Q. (2018). Ketamine in electroconvulsive therapy for depressive disorder: A systematic review and meta-analysis. Journal of Psychiatric Research, 104, 144–156. https://doi.org/10.1016/j.jpsychires.2018.07.003

Réus, G. Z., Abelaira, H. M., dos Santos, M. A. B., Carlessi, A. S., Tomaz, D. B., Neotti, M. V., Liranço, J. L. G., Gubert, C., Barth, M., Kapczinski, F., & Quevedo, J. (2013). Ketamine and imipramine in the nucleus accumbens regulate histone deacetylation induced by maternal deprivation and are critical for associated behaviors. Behavioural Brain Research, 256, 451–456. https://doi.org/10.1016/j. bbr.2013.08.041

Ricke, A. K., Snook, R. J., & Anand, A. (2011). Induction of Prolonged Mania During Ketamine Therapy for Reflex Sympathetic Dystrophy. Biological Psychiatry, 70(4), e13–e14. https://doi.org/10.1016/j.biopsych.2011.02.030

Rodrigues, N. B., McIntyre, R. S., Lipsitz, O., Lee, Y., Cha, D. S., Nasri, F., Gill, H., Lui, L. M. W., Subramaniapillai, M., Kratiuk, K., Lin, K., Ho, R., Mansur, R. B., & Rosenblat, J. D. (2020). Safety and tolerability of IV ketamine in adults with major depressive or bipolar disorder: results from the Canadian rapid treatment center of excellence. Expert Opinion on Drug Safety, 19(8), 1031–1040. https://doi.org/10.1080/14740338.2020.1776699

Rodriguez, C. I., Kegeles, L. S., Flood, P., & Simpson, H. B. (2011). Rapid Resolution of Obsessions After an Infusion of Intravenous Ketamine in a Patient With Treatment-Resistant Obsessive-Compulsive Disorder. The Journal of Clinical Psychiatry, 72(04), 567–569. https://doi.org/10.4088/jcp.10l06653

Rodriguez, C. I., Kegeles, L. S., Levinson, A., Feng, T., Marcus, S. M., Vermes, D., Flood, P., & Simpson, H. B. (2013). Randomized Controlled Crossover Trial of Ketamine in Obsessive-Compulsive Disorder: Proof-of-Concept. Neuropsychopharmacology, 38(12), 2475–2483. https://doi.org/10.1038/npp.2013.150

Rodriguez, C. I., Kegeles, L. S., Levinson, A., Ogden, R. T., Mao, X., Milak, M. S., Vermes, D., Xie, S., Hunter, L., Flood, P., Moore, H., Shungu, D. C., & Simpson, H. B. (2015). In vivo effects of ketamine on glutamate-glutamine and gamma-aminobutyric acid in obsessive-compulsive disorder: Proof of concept. Psychiatry Research: Neuroimaging, 233(2), 141–147. https://doi.org/10.1016/j.pscychresns.2015.06.001

Rodriguez, C. I., Lapidus, K. A. B., Zwerling, J., Levinson, A., Mahnke, A., Steinman, S. A., Kalanthroff, E., & Simpson, H. B.

(2017). Challenges in Testing Intranasal Ketamine in Obsessive-Compulsive Disorder. The Journal of Clinical Psychiatry, 78(04), 466–467. https://doi.org/10.4088/jcp.16cr11234

Rush, A. J. (2013). Ketamine for Treatment-Resistant Depression: Ready or Not for Clinical Use? American Journal of Psychiatry, 170(10), 1079–1081. https://doi.org/10.1176/appi.ajp.2013.13081034

Rybakowski, J. K., Permoda-Osip, A., & Bartkowska-Sniatkowska, A. (2017). Ketamine augmentation rapidly improves depression scores in inpatients with treatment-resistant bipolar depression. International Journal of Psychiatry in Clinical Practice, 21(2), 99–103. https://doi.org/10.1080/13651501.2017.1297834

S Correia-Melo, F., C Argolo, F., Araújo-de-Freitas, L., Carneiro Gomes Leal, G., Kapczinski, F., L Lacerda, A., & C Quarantini, L. (2017). Rapid infusion of esketamine for unipolar and bipolar depression: a retrospective chart review. Neuropsychiatric Disease and Treatment, Volume 13, 1627–1632. https://doi.org/10.2147/ndt.s135623

SAMHSA. (2022, May 14). National Helpline | SAMHSA - Substance Abuse and Mental Health Services Administration. Samhsa.gov. https://www.samhsa.gov/find-help/national-helpline

Schaffer, A., Isometsä, E. T., Tondo, L., H Moreno, D., Turecki, G., Reis, C., Cassidy, F., Sinyor, M., Azorin, J.-M., Kessing, L. V., Ha, K., Goldstein, T., Weizman, A., Beautrais, A., Chou, Y.-H., Diazgranados, N., Levitt, A. J., Zarate, C. A., Rihmer, Z., & Yatham, L. N. (2014). International Society for Bipolar Disorders Task Force on Suicide: meta-analyses and meta-regression of correlates of suicide attempts and suicide deaths in bipolar disorder. Bipolar Disorders, 17(1), 1–16. https://doi.org/10.1111/bdi.12271

Schatzberg, A. F. (2014). A Word to the Wise About Ketamine.

American Journal of Psychiatry, 171(3), 262–264. https://doi.org/10. 1176/appi.ajp.2014.13101434

Schwartz, J., Murrough, J. W., & Iosifescu, D. V. (2016). Ketamine for treatment-resistant depression: recent developments and clinical applications. Evidence-Based Mental Health, 19(2), 35–38. https://doi.org/10.1136/eb-2016-102355

Serafini, G., Howland, R., Rovedi, F., Girardi, P., & Amore, M. (2014). The Role of Ketamine in Treatment-Resistant Depression: A Systematic Review. Current Neuropharmacology, 12(5), 444–461. https://doi.org/10.2174/1570159x12666140619204251

Shaw, S. (2022, June 6). What These Patient Advocates Want You to Know About Migraine. GHLF.org. https://ghlf.org/migraine/what-these-patient-advocates-want-you-to-know-about-migraine/

Shi, J., Badner, J. A., Hattori, E., Potash, J. B., Willour, V. L., McMahon, F. J., Gershon, E. S., & Liu, C. (2008). Neurotransmission and bipolar disorder: A systematic family-based association study. American Journal of Medical Genetics Part B: Neuropsychiatric Genetics, 147B(7), 1270–1277. https://doi.org/10.1002/ajmg.b.30769

Short, B., Fong, J., Galvez, V., Shelker, W., & Loo, C. K. (2018). Side-effects associated with ketamine use in depression: a systematic review. The Lancet Psychiatry, 5(1), 65–78. https://doi.org/10.1016/ s2215-0366(17)30272-9

Shteamer, J. W., Callaway, M. A., Patel, P., & Singh, V. (2019). How effective is ketamine in the management of chronic neuropathic pain? Pain Management, 9(6), 517–519. https://doi.org/10.2217/pmt-2019-0032

Singh-Manoux, A., Dugravot, A., Fournier, A., Abell, J., Ebmeier, K., Kivimäki, M., & Sabia, S. (2017). Trajectories of Depressive

Symptoms Before Diagnosis of Dementia. JAMA Psychiatry, 74(7), 712–718. https://doi.org/10.1001/jamapsychiatry.2017.0660

Sinner, B., & Graf, B. M. (2008). Ketamine. Handbook of Experimental Pharmacology, 182, 313–333. https://doi.org/10.1007/978-3-540-74806-9_15

Smalheiser, N. R. (2019). Ketamine: A Neglected Therapy for Alzheimer Disease. Frontiers in Aging Neuroscience, 11. https://doi.org/10.3389/fnagi.2019.00186

Smith-Apeldoorn, S. Y., Veraart, J. K. E., Kamphuis, J., van Asselt, A. D. I., Touw, D. J., aan het Rot, M., & Schoevers, R. A. (2019). Oral esketamine for treatment-resistant depression: rationale and design of a randomized controlled trial. BMC Psychiatry, 19(1). https://doi.org/10.1186/s12888-019-2359-1

Spottswood, M., Davydow, D. S., & Huang, H. (2017). The Prevalence of Posttraumatic Stress Disorder in Primary Care. Harvard Review of Psychiatry, 25(4), 1. https://doi.org/10.1097/hrp.0000000000000136

Staff, E. (n.d.). Physical Symptoms of Ketamine Abuse: Short-Term & Physiological Effects. American Addiction Centers. https://americanaddictioncenters.org/ketamine-abuse/physical-symptoms

Substance Abuse and Mental Health Services Administration. (2016). Table 3.13, DSM-IV to DSM-5 Obsessive-Compulsive Disorder Comparison. Nih.gov; Substance Abuse and Mental Health Services Administration (US). https://www.ncbi.nlm.nih.gov/books/NBK519704/table/ch3.t13/

Suicidal Ideation: Symptoms, Finding Help, and More. (n.d.). Healthline. https://www.healthline.com/health/suicidal-ideation

Suleiman, Z., Ik, K., & Bo, B. (2012). Evaluation of the cardiovascular stimulation effects after induction of anaesthesia with ketamine. Journal of the West African College of Surgeons, 2(1), 38–52. https://europepmc.org/article/MED/25452977

Swedo, S. E., Schrag, A., Gilbert, R., Giovannoni, G., Robertson, M. M., Metcalfe, C., Ben-Shlomo, Y., & Gilbert, D. L. (2010). STREP-TOCOCCAL INFECTION, TOURETTE SYNDROME, AND OCD: IS THERE A CONNECTION? PANDAS: HORSE OR ZEBRA? Neurology, 74(17), 1397–1399. https://doi.org/10.1212/wnl.0b013e3181d8a638

Sy Jye Leu, Yang, Y., Hsing Cheng Liu, Cheng, C.-Y., Wu, Y., Huang, M.-C., Lee, Y.-L., Chen, C.-C., Shen, W.-D., & Liu, K.-J. (2017). Valproic Acid and Lithium Mediate Anti-Inflammatory Effects by Differentially Modulating Dendritic Cell Differentiation and Function. Journal of Cellular Physiology, 232(5), 1176–1186. https://doi.org/10.1002/jcp.25604

The 6 Best Chronic Pain Support Groups of 2021. (n.d.). Verywell Health. https://www.verywellhealth.com/best-chronic-pain-support-groups-4845866

The Facts About Migraine. (n.d.). American Migraine Foundation. Retrieved October 23, 2023, from https://americanmigrainefoundation.org/resource-library/facts-about-migraine/

The Ketamine Clinic Craze: Legalities and Possibilities. (2020, March 4). Harris Sliwoski LLP (Formerly Harris Bricken). http://harrisbricken.com/cannalawblog/the-ketamine-clinic-craze-legalities-and-possibilities/

There are 3 Types of Ketamine—Which One Works Best? (2020, May 18). DoubleBlind Mag. https://doubleblindmag.com/there-are-3-types-of-ketamine-which-one-works-best/

Turek, Melissa. "Creating a Therapeutic Environment to Improve Outcomes with Ketamine Infusion Therapy." 2023.

FRANK M LIGONS

Turna, J., Grosman Kaplan, K., Anglin, R., & Van Ameringen, M. (2015). "WHAT'S BUGGING THE GUT IN OCD?" A REVIEW OF THE GUT MICROBIOME IN OBSESSIVE-COMPULSIVE DISORDER. Depression and Anxiety, 33(3), 171–178. https://doi.org/10.1002/da.22454

Uemura, K., Shimada, H., Doi, T., Makizako, H., Park, H., & Suzuki, T. (2014). Depressive symptoms in older adults are associated with decreased cerebral oxygenation of the prefrontal cortex during a trail-making test. Archives of Gerontology and Geriatrics, 59(2), 422–428. https://doi.org/10.1016/j.archger.2014.07.003

Uguz, F., Akman, C., Kaya, N., & Cilli, A. S. (2007). Postpartum-Onset Obsessive-Compulsive Disorder. The Journal of Clinical Psychiatry, 68(01), 132–138. https://doi.org/10.4088/jcp.v68n0118

UpToDate. (n.d.). Www.uptodate.com. https://www.uptodate.com/contents/ketamine-and-esketamine-for-treating-unipolar-depression-in-adults-administration-efficacy-and-adverse-effects

VA.gov | Veterans Affairs. (2017). Va.gov. https://www.healthquality.va.gov/guidelines/MH/ptsd/

Varghese, M., & Muliyala, K. (2010). The complex relationship between depression and dementia. Annals of Indian Academy of Neurology, 13(6), 69. https://doi.org/10.4103/0972-2327.74248

Volkow, N. D., & Li, T.-K. (2004). Drug addiction: the neurobiology of behaviour gone awry. Nature Reviews Neuroscience, 5(12), 963–970. https://doi.org/10.1038/nrn1539

Wan, L.-B., Levitch, C. F., Perez, A. M., Brallier, J. W., Iosifescu, D. V., Chang, L. C., Foulkes, A., Mathew, S. J., Charney, D. S., & Murrough, J. W. (2014). Ketamine Safety and Tolerability in Clinical Trials for Treatment-Resistant Depression. The Journal of

Clinical Psychiatry, 76(03), 247–252. https://doi.org/10.4088/jcp. 13m08852

Wang, A. K., & Miller, B. J. (2017). Meta-analysis of Cerebrospinal Fluid Cytokine and Tryptophan Catabolite Alterations in Psychiatric Patients: Comparisons Between Schizophrenia, Bipolar Disorder, and Depression. Schizophrenia Bulletin, 44(1), 75–83. https://doi.org/10.1093/schbul/sbx035

Wei, Y., Chang, L., & Hashimoto, K. (2020). A historical review of antidepressant effects of ketamine and its enantiomers. Pharmacology Biochemistry and Behavior, 190, 172870. https://doi.org/10. 1016/j.pbb.2020.172870

What Is Dementia? (2020). Alzheimer's Disease and Dementia. https://www.alz.org/alzheimers-dementia/what-is-demen tia#:~:text=What%20Is%20Dementia%3F-

WHITE, J. M., & RYAN, C. F. (1996). Pharmacological properties of ketamine. Drug and Alcohol Review, 15(2), 145–155. https://doi.org/ 10.1080/09595239600185801

White, P. F., Ham, J., Way, W. L., & Trevor, A. (1980). Pharmacology of Ketamine Isomers in Surgical Patients. Anesthesiology, 52(3), 231–239. https://doi.org/10.1097/00000542-198003000-00008

White, T. (2017, August 17). The pros and cons of ketamine for obsessive compulsive disorder (OCD). Stanford Medicine Magazine. http://stanmed.stanford.edu/2017summer/carolyn-rodriguez-ketamine-OCD.html

Wilkinson, S. T., Ballard, E. D., Bloch, M. H., Mathew, S. J., Murrough, J. W., Feder, A., Sos, P., Wang, G., Zarate, C. A., & Sanacora, G. (2018). The Effect of a Single Dose of Intravenous Ketamine on Suicidal Ideation: A Systematic Review and Individual

Participant Data Meta-Analysis. The American Journal of Psychiatry, 175(2), 150–158. https://doi.org/10.1176/appi.ajp.2017.17040472

Wilkowska, A., Szałach, Ł. P., & Cubała, W. J. (2021). Gut Microbiota in Depression: A Focus on Ketamine. Frontiers in Behavioral Neuroscience, 15, 693362. https://doi.org/10.3389/fnbeh.2021.693362

Wilkowska, A., Szałach, Ł., & Cubała, W. J. (2020). Ketamine in Bipolar Disorder: A Review. Neuropsychiatric Disease and Treatment, Volume 16, 2707–2717. https://doi.org/10.2147/ndt.s282208

Wilkowska, A., Szałach, Ł., Słupski, J., Wielewicka, A., Czarnota, M., Gałuszko-Węgielnik, M., Wiglusz, M. S., & Cubała, W. J. (2020). Affective Switch Associated With Oral, Low Dose Ketamine Treatment in a Patient With Treatment Resistant Bipolar I Depression. Case Report and Literature Review. Frontiers in Psychiatry, 11. https://doi.org/10.3389/fpsyt.2020.00516

Woelfer, M., Li, M., Colic, L., Liebe, T., Di, X., Biswal, B., Murrough, J., Lessmann, V., Brigadski, T., & Walter, M. (2019). Ketamine-induced changes in plasma brain-derived neurotrophic factor (BDNF) levels are associated with the resting-state functional connectivity of the prefrontal cortex. The World Journal of Biological Psychiatry, 1–15. https://doi.org/10.1080/15622975.2019.1679391

Wong, A., Benedict, N. J., Armahizer, M. J., & Kane-Gill, S. L. (2015). Evaluation of adjunctive ketamine to benzodiazepines for management of alcohol withdrawal syndrome. The Annals of Pharmacotherapy, 49(1), 14–19. https://doi.org/10.1177/1060028014555859

Xu, Y., Hackett, M., Carter, G., Loo, C., Gálvez, V., Glozier, N., Glue, P., Lapidus, K., McGirr, A., Somogyi, A. A., Mitchell, P. B., & Rodgers, A. (2015). Effects of Low-Dose and Very Low-Dose Ketamine among Patients with Major Depression: a Systematic

Review and Meta-Analysis. International Journal of Neuropsychopharmacology, 19(4), pyv124. https://doi.org/10.1093/ijnp/pyv124

Yang, C., Shirayama, Y., Zhang, J-c., Ren, Q., Yao, W., Ma, M., Dong, C., & Hashimoto, K. (2015). R-ketamine: a rapid-onset and sustained antidepressant without psychotomimetic side effects. Translational Psychiatry, 5(9), e632–e632. https://doi.org/10.1038/tp.2015.136

Zanos, P., & Gould, T. D. (2018). Mechanisms of ketamine action as an antidepressant. Molecular Psychiatry, 23(4), 801–811. https://doi.org/10.1038/mp.2017.255

Zanos, P., Moaddel, R., Morris, P. J., Georgiou, P., Fischell, J., Elmer, G. I., Alkondon, M., Yuan, P., Pribut, H. J., Singh, N. S., Dossou, K. S. S., Fang, Y., Huang, X.-P., Mayo, C. L., Wainer, I. W., Albuquerque, E. X., Thompson, S. M., Thomas, C. J., Zarate Jr, C. A., & Gould, T. D. (2016). NMDAR inhibition-independent antidepressant actions of ketamine metabolites. Nature, 533(7604), 481–486. https://doi.org/10.1038/nature17998

Zarate, C. A., Brutsche, N. E., Ibrahim, L., Franco-Chaves, J., Diazgranados, N., Cravchik, A., Selter, J., Marquardt, C. A., Liberty, V., & Luckenbaugh, D. A. (2012). Replication of Ketamine's Antidepressant Efficacy in Bipolar Depression: A Randomized Controlled Add-On Trial. Biological Psychiatry, 71(11), 939–946. https://doi.org/10.1016/j.biopsych.2011.12.010

Zarate, C. A., Singh, J., & Manji, H. K. (2006). Cellular Plasticity Cascades: Targets for the Development of Novel Therapeutics for Bipolar Disorder. Biological Psychiatry, 59(11), 1006–1020. https://doi.org/10.1016/j.biopsych.2005.10.021

Zhang, J., Li, S., & Hashimoto, K. (2014). R (–)-ketamine shows greater potency and longer lasting antidepressant effects than S

(+)-ketamine. Pharmacology Biochemistry and Behavior, 116, 137–141. https://doi.org/10.1016/j.pbb.2013.11.033

Zhao, M., Wang, W., Jiang, Z., Zhu, Z., Liu, D., & Pan, F. (2020). Long-Term Effect of Post-traumatic Stress in Adolescence on Dendrite Development and H3K9me2/BDNF Expression in Male Rat Hippocampus and Prefrontal Cortex. Frontiers in Cell and Developmental Biology, 8. https://doi.org/10.3389/fcell.2020.00682

Zheng, P., Zeng, B., Zhou, C., Liu, M., Fang, Z., Xu, X., Zeng, L., Chen, J., Fan, S., Du, X., Zhang, X., Yang, D., Yang, Y., Meng, H., Li, W., Melgiri, N. D., Licinio, J., Wei, H., & Xie, P. (2016). Gut microbiome remodeling induces depressive-like behaviors through a pathway mediated by the host's metabolism. Molecular Psychiatry, 21(6), 786–796. https://doi.org/10.1038/mp.2016.44

Zheng, W., Zhou, Y.-L., Liu, W.-J., Wang, C.-Y., Zhan, Y.-N., Lan, X.-F., Zhang, B., & Ning, Y.-P. (2020). A preliminary study of adjunctive ketamine for treatment-resistant bipolar depression. Journal of Affective Disorders, 275, 38–43. https://doi.org/10.1016/j.jad.2020.06.020

Zhou, Y., & Danbolt, N. C. (2014). Glutamate as a neurotransmitter in the healthy brain. Journal of Neural Transmission, 121(8), 799–817. https://doi.org/10.1007/s00702-014-1180-8

Zimmerman, J. M., & Maren, S. (2010). NMDA receptor antagonism in the basolateral but not central amygdala blocks the extinction of Pavlovian fear conditioning in rats. European Journal of Neuroscience, no-no. https://doi.org/10.1111/j.1460-9568.2010.07223.x

Zorumski, C. F., Izumi, Y., & Mennerick, S. (2016). Ketamine: NMDA Receptors and Beyond. The Journal of Neuroscience, 36(44), 11158–11164. https://doi.org/10.1523/jneurosci.1547-16.2016